To
Lose Weight
Change Shape

Body-Shaping the **TLC** Way
– The Plan That *Really* Works

Janet Thomson

Thorsons
An Imprint of HarperCollins*Publishers*

Thorsons
An Imprint of HarperCollins*Publishers*
77–85 Fulham Palace Road
Hammersmith, London W6 8JB
1160 Battery Street
San Francisco, California 94111–1213

Published by Thorsons 1996
1 3 5 7 9 10 8 6 4 2

A catalogue record for this book
is available from the British Library

ISBN 0 7225 3355 1

Text illustrations by Andrea Norton

Printed and bound in Great Britain by
Caledonian International Book Manufacturing Ltd, Glasgow

Contents

This book is dedicated to my husband Laurie for putting up with me for the last 15 years (not easy!) and my wonderful children, Ben 13, Ryan 11, and Emilie 6, who are a constant source of joy. Thanks to Ian Uttley for the inspirational title, and to Dian Mills at the Institute of Optimum Nutrition for being a patient tutor when I couldn't hand my assignments in on time – and for her invaluable help with designing the recipies (and to my family for trying them out!) Thanks also to Wanda Whiteley and Cresta Norris at HarperCollins for looking after me so well and for their continued support.

Introduction

Are you happy with the shape of your body or would you like to change it? If you are reading this book, you probably want to change it. Most of us would like to tone up, lose weight and change shape, but don't know how to do it.

So what makes this book different from all the other so-called 'weight loss' and 'diet' books you may have seen? The answer is: it works, it's easy to follow and the results are long term. It really will show you how to change your shape and lose body fat – and keep it off for good. You will understand how and why it works as you read the book. I will explain to you how you really can lose weight safely and effectively, have more energy and feel great.

There are no gimmicks, no quick fix cures, just easy to follow advice. Once you know how you store body fat and what makes you into an 'apple' or a 'pear' shape, you can change that shape. Of course we all inherit a blueprint – a genetic make up that dictates what shape we will be – but more often than not this shape becomes exaggerated when we gain weight. In other words, you may have a pear-shaped figure when you are overweight, but when you lose the excess fat and tone up certain parts of the body, it is hardly noticeable!

You will learn all about fat – are all fats equal?

Certainly not, and you will see why.

If you have read my first book, *Fat to Flat* (Thorsons, 1995), then you will already know how the body can be trained to burn fat more efficiently. Have you ever wondered why you get hungry and if it really is possible to train your appetite so that you only want to eat the foods that you should eat and avoid cravings? Yes it is possible and I'll show you how.

Find out which foods speed up your metabolism or slow it down and which fats you need and which you should avoid. There is also advice on choosing clothes and styles that flatter your figure and you can select the exercise programme specifically designed for your body shape.

You may read the book from cover to cover in one go or you may pick it up and put it down. You will find that it is divided into sections or topics, which makes it easier to 'dip into' from time to time. Either way, you will learn everything you need to know about how to lose weight and achieve the shape that you want.

I wish you every success. Only *you* have the power to change your shape – go for it!

Part 1: Be Prepared

Chapter 1

Are You Ready for This?

Your body won't suddenly change by itself – you have to make it happen. In order for you to be successful at losing weight and improving your body shape, you have to be ready to make the necessary changes. After all, if you carry on as you are, i.e. doing the things that have caused you to become overweight, common sense will tell you that you will continue to become more overweight. In this section I will give you methods that you can use to motivate yourself and monitor your progress. After all, you want to see and feel the results.

It is really helpful to have a stage of pondering or preparing before embarking on a new programme. In order to do this and to help you in the future, I want you to write down everything you eat and drink for the next three days, *before* you start the recipes or exercise programmes in the book. This may sound like a strange thing to do, as many of you will be chomping at the bit and just want to get started right away – but believe me, it will be very beneficial in times to come.

It is important that you eat just as you have done in the past. If you don't eat things because you would have to write them down, it won't be accurate.

Use the chart overleaf – either photocopy it or

write one out for yourself. You will need several copies.

At the top of each page put the date. Use a separate sheet for each day. Next, log the time you are eating. Make sure you fill this in *at the time of eating,* not at the end of the day. Then fill in the place. This is important when it comes to planning your food in the future – it will enable you to identify situations when you are at 'high risk' of either overeating generally or of making the wrong choices in terms of snacks.

Place a tick or a cross in the column that asks whether the food was pre-planned or not. One of the most important things you must do is to learn to plan your meals *and* your snacks. It is important you do not feel hungry – after all, this is not a short-term four-week diet that you will give up as soon as you have finished, it is learning how to develop positive eating habits that you will be able to maintain in the long term. It is about permanent change for the good.

In the column that asks how you feel after the food, write down whether you feel you have overeaten or have eaten about the right amount. Also note whether the food was positive or negative, i.e. whether it will help you to lose weight or to gain weight. Write down whether you feel good or bad after eating your food. How many times have you eaten something that you didn't really want, just because it looked or smelled good, and regretted it afterwards? Recognizing the foods that make you feel like this will help you to stop eating them.

Table 1:

Date	
Time	
Food or Drink	
Place	
Pre-planned Y/N	
Feeling/Mood e.g. happy/bored	
How You Felt Afterwards e.g. was it excessive or OK	
Exercise Y/N	

PLANNING AHEAD

Three meals per day are essential. Breakfast is crucial as it will get your metabolism going for the day. Even if you only have time for some fruit, you must have something to see you through the morning and prevent snacking.

Lunch must also be pre-planned, particularly if you work and often find yourself in the delicatessen grabbing a cheese sandwich and a packet of crisps or a bun. Instead, you should get into the habit of making your own lunch to take with you. You don't have to stick to sandwiches – in fact I don't recommend having large amounts of bread every day, as this can lead to abdominal bloating and bowel irregularity *(see page 52)*. So, if you are already having toast for breakfast, try to choose something other than bread for lunch. During the winter I have home-made soups most days *(see the recipe section)*. These freeze really well and can be taken in a flask if you don't have any heating facilities at work. I also take rye crisp breads, which dunk in soup surprisingly well. If you do have sandwiches, see the suggested fillings on page 170. I suggest you also have a piece of fruit or a low-fat yoghurt. You must feel satisfied, otherwise you will be tempted to pick or snack all afternoon.

Your evening meal must also be pre-planned, as this prevents the temptation to call in at the nearest takeaway or fast food restaurant on the way home. If you work full time, a slow cooker is a must. Before you go out, you can put in a selection of vegetables and some spices, a tin of tomatoes and a small amount of the meat of your choice (lean cuts only and preferably white meat), or beans and lentils, and you will come home to a beautifully cooked, delicious meal. You have only to boil some rice or some potatoes and it is ready.

Other quick and easy alternatives are stir fries, which can be prepared and cooked in about 15 minutes. Try to make the majority of the stir fry vegetables. Carrots, baby sweetcorn, sugar snaps, mangetout, celery, peppers, small broccoli or cauliflower florets all stir fry really well and stay nice and crisp if you only cook them for a few minutes. For the meat, I suggest two chicken fillets to serve four people, served with loads of vegetables or beans. Add some soy sauce or other seasoning to taste. I sometimes use jars of ready-made sauce. The sweet and sour variety, for example, is lovely – you just pour it over the ingredients as you stir and it's ready in minutes. Check the labels, though, for large amounts of sugar. Some varieties do a 'light' alternative which is lower in sugar.

You must also pre-plan your snacks. Eating between meals is OK as long as you monitor what you eat and don't snack on chocolate, biscuits, crisps or other high-fat 'negative' foods. Such foods are just empty calories. This means although they are high in calories, they are empty of nutrients. Fruit is probably the best snack food, particularly if you are out and about or at work and you have to take it with you. Try and vary the fruit you eat – don't always stick to apples, for example. It is always a good idea to go for whatever fruit is in season. You should have three pieces of fruit per day, in addition to any with your meals: one mid-morning, one mid-afternoon and one in the evening.

If you are at home, then raw vegetables make a great snack. You can have these with a low-fat dip *(see the recipe for hummus on page 171)*. Most supermarkets sell low-fat fromage frais dips, which are lovely, but always check the label before you buy and go for a fat content of 4 g per 100 g (0.1 oz per 3.5 oz) or less. You could also try guacamole, tofu dips or taramasalata if they are low fat.

WHAT ARE YOU GOING TO EAT NEXT?

At any time of the day or evening, you must know exactly when and what you are going to eat next. Erratic eating patterns disrupt the body's normal sensations of hunger *(see page 38 for more about hunger and appetite)* and if you plan what you are going to eat, it helps to resist the urge to overeat on negative foods.

Meals and snacks are like stepping-stones that get you through the day. Eating three meals per day and fruit or healthy snacks in between will not cause you to gain weight, it will cause you to *lose* weight at a steady rate and will nourish your body. If, on the other hand, you eat high-calorie, low-nutrient foods such as sweets, cakes, etc., then although you have given your body adequate calories, it will still crave food in an attempt to get you to eat something nutritious. People often try to satisfy this urge to eat with more sweets or refined, i.e. highly processed, foods. The problem with these foods is that the refining process removes most of the vitamins and minerals contained in the foods in their natural state. So you end up in a never-ending circle of food cravings being satisfied with poor quality foods. There is a large percentage of the Western population walking around today regularly consuming more calories than they need, but lacking many essential nutrients. If this happens, you are also more likely to suffer from stress and other diseases, as some of the body's vital organs and systems are not getting the nutrients they need in order to function properly.

NOT EVERYONE'S PERFECT!

Once you are on the plan, don't feel bad if you slip up now and then. Give yourself time. After all, you have become so used to the way you eat that permanent change may seem impossible. It isn't. You may just need a little time to implement your new pattern of eating. Remember, there is a big difference between a lapse, which is a temporary slip, and a relapse, which is a return to your previous habits. You don't have to turn a lapse into a relapse. I have been changing my eating habits for the past two years and I am still improving my diet.

It is unlikely that you are going to change your eating habits so dramatically in one swoop that you never eat anything you feel you shouldn't again. The joy of this eating plan is that once you have got used to changing the balance of what you eat, i.e. eating less meat and fewer dairy products and eating more vegetable and plant based foods, the *occasional* piece of chocolate cake won't make any difference. Whilst you are getting used to changing your eating habits, you should expect the occasional slip and not punish yourself. Rest assured that it is quite normal and needn't be a problem as long as you recognize it for what it is.

Of course I am not suggesting that you have a bar

of chocolate any time you feel hungry – you should try to re-educate your palate by choosing something else! What I am saying, however, is that if you feel that you have 'failed' by eating something you shouldn't, then you are likely to stop trying altogether. If this happens, not only will you not lose weight, but you may even actually eat more in attempt to cheer yourself up and *gain* weight. This need not be the case. You will find that as you get used to your new eating habits, these small lapses become fewer.

It will also take time for you to find other alternatives to some of the foods you have been eating up until now. But once you have replaced the high-calorie, high-fat foods with something that is more nutritious, you will find it much easier.

ONE STEP AT A TIME

If, once you have read this book, you feel ready to make some changes but don't want to do it all at once, give yourself one goal per month. For example, in the first month aim to eat more vegetables with every meal. This means adding more vegetables to your favourite dishes as well as serving more vegetables with your meal. In the second month try to reduce the amount of meat you eat, in particular red meat. You must also take into account how your new way of eating will affect your family or other people that you may cook for or share meals with.

Try introducing some beans or lentils to your meals. When someone first suggested using lentils to me I didn't know what to do with them. I thought it meant hours of soaking and washing them before

I could use them, and with three children to feed and working full time, I didn't feel I could fit it in. In reality, I now buy a box of red lentils, which only need to be boiled for about 20 minutes (see instructions on packet), and add them to whatever I am making. I started off by adding them to shepherd's pie, a favourite with the children. They didn't even notice! My shepherd's pie is now made up of mashed root vegetables such as swede and carrots, lentils and a little turkey mince. The mashed potato on the top is cooked and mashed with parsnips. This makes a really well balanced meal, but at the same time, it is an old favourite that they are used to. I have just changed the way I cook it. I have also been able to add lentils to casseroles, curries and stews in the same way.

THINK AHEAD

Noting the mood you are in before you eat is also very important, as it helps to identify 'triggers' that affect your eating behaviour. For example, if you are eating because you are bored, then you will be able to identify these moments as 'high risk' and prepare for them so that you do not grab the first high-calorie food that you see, which is often chocolate or cheese and biscuits. Research has suggested that people who are overweight often consume more calories from snack foods than they do from meals. This might sound a little unbelievable, but when you consider you can have a delicious meal of vegetables and a little meat in a tomato and herb sauce with some rice all for the same amount of calories you might consume in a large bar of chocolate, it becomes a little easier to understand. You would probably be unpleasantly surprised if you added up the calorific value of all the snack foods you regularly eat!

As already explained, if you are eating because you are bored, planning your snacks can go a long way to overcoming the problem. This way you do not feel deprived – you simply make different choices.

THE POSITIVE APPROACH

Learning to identify foods as positive or negative will help you to make the right choices in the future. If a food is plant based, then it is definitely positive. Plant based foods are carbohydrates *(see page 43 for more information)*. They will provide your body with the maximum amount of nutrients and will help to stimulate your metabolism without causing you to gain excess weight.

Hard cheese and large amounts of meat are definitely negative foods. (A small amount of meat is fine, but a steak or a burger, for example, is not.) Always remember the age-old saying – prevention is better than cure. It only takes two or three minutes of will-power to resist, but may take hours and hours of exercise to remove! The choice is yours.

ADD IT ALL UP

When you have completed the three days, look first at the total amount you have eaten. People are often surprised at how much they actually eat. When you really write down every biscuit or nibble of cheese, it can be quite alarming. But be honest with yourself, then you will achieve your goals.

Look at the content of the food you have eaten and see if you can work out what approximate percentage was carbohydrate, i.e. organic plant based foods, and what was fat or protein based, i.e. animal foods, including dairy products. (I have put fat and protein together here to simplify it as much as possible.) To lose weight and keep it off, you need to make sure that the majority of your foods are carbohydrates. You will learn more about carbohydrate, fat and protein later on and will soon be able to identify which is which very easily.

Look at everything you have eaten during the day and write 'C' by carbohydrate foods and 'FP' by fat or protein foods. Fat contains twice as many calories per gram as carbohydrate, so multiply the number of FPs by 2 and then add up the number of Cs. The ideal would be 60–70 per cent C to 20–30 per cent FP.

Table 2 is a typical example taken from a member of my club. As you can see, she only just managed to get her carbohydrate level above the fat level on this day. I have allowed one C for each portion of carbohydrate, for example for breakfast she had a C for the grapefruit and a C for the cereals. For lunch she had FP for the fat and protein in the pâté (which is a very high-fat food), and a C for the bread. For dinner she had C for the pasta, FP for the chicken and C for the vegetables.

My advice for this day was to leave breakfast as it is and perhaps have a piece of fruit during the morning. For lunch, almost anything is better in a sandwich than pâté, so a different filling such as tuna salad would be preferable. Dinner is fine, except that she could have had two portions of vegetables instead

Table 2:

Date	18.1	
Breakfast	2 cups tea ½ grapefruit bran flakes & raisins	C C
Lunch	pâté sandwich coffee	FP C
Dinner	chicken pasta & veg. cup of tea	C FP C
Extras	none	
	Total FP 2 x 2 = 4	C 5

of one. Had she done this, then her carbohydrate to fat and protein ratio would have been much better.

You will probably also find that at the moment you are eating too much fat and protein. Writing down everything you eat and evaluating it in this way will help you to achieve the right balance. It is only a very rough guide and doesn't accurately take into account quantities, but I have used it very successfully with many people and it has really made them analyse what they are eating. It also shows that if you have one slip up it doesn't change the whole balance – but if you have lots of them it definitely does.

Remember, the aim is to achieve a mainly carbohydrate based diet, made up of lots of vegetables and fruit and natural whole foods, and less meat, dairy produce and refined or processed foods. Nature provides us with all the foods we need to eat to stay healthy without becoming overweight.

MAKE A NOTE

When you start the diet in this book, log what you eat in exactly the same way and watch the balance start to change. If you follow the recipes exactly, including three or more pieces of fruit per day, you can rest assured you will be getting it right. If you are following your own recipes, then you need to adapt them so that you increase the amount of vegetables and decrease the amount of meat. If you are having too much fat and protein, you will find all the information you need to redress the balance in the following chapters.

If you are a vegetarian, you may need to look at

dairy products such as cheese, which is very high in saturated fat. Many vegetarian meals rely heavily on cheese, rather than on the vegetables themselves. Nuts are also used in many vegetarian recipes and whilst a few daily can be a good source of essential fatty acids *(see pp. 67–74)*, too many can lead to weight gain.

You may be thinking that you don't have the time to write everything down, but you must make time. You may only need to do it for a couple of weeks, until getting the right balance has become a habit. If at the end of each day you have achieved 60 per cent or more carbohydrate to fat and protein ratio, then you are well on your way to losing weight and keeping it off. Then it is useful to do a log every once in a while, just for a day, to make sure you are staying on the right track.

If you begin to struggle or to regain weight at any point, start writing down what you eat in the same way. This will help you to find out where you are going wrong and help you to put things right.

YOU *CAN* DO IT!

If you are unhappy about being overweight, you must face up to the fact that you *do* have the power to change – permanently. But you will need to organize and plan your food for a while until you develop new habits. When you are automatically making positive choices, you won't need to think about it any more – it will have become a way of life. So will being slimmer and feeling great! If you follow this programme, you really will tone up, lose weight and change shape – for good.

CHECK YOUR PROGRESS

After a few weeks, you will be able to see and feel the difference. You must remember that 1 lb (0.4 kg) of body fat takes up more space on your body than 1 lb of muscle, so don't worry if you are not losing as much as you would like on the scales. It is far better to judge how you look, and watch your measurements and your shape start to change. You could use some clothes that are a little tight and try them on every week to see when they become loose again, or you could just record your measurements. If you do this, I suggest you keep a monthly record as shown in the table on page 16.

Take your measurements before you start the plan. You may find it easier to get someone to help you. You must make sure you measure in exactly the same place each time. For the upper arm you could put on a short-sleeved T-shirt and measure at the end of the sleeve. For the individual thighs you could use a pair of shorts and roll them up to the widest point. Keep them rolled up and just use them when you are measuring.

HOW QUICKLY WILL I LOSE WEIGHT?

You will probably start to see a reduction within three to four weeks, but everyone is different. You must allow your body time to make the adjustments. Remember, it takes the body a long time to burn 1 lb (0.4 kg) of fat. It represents 3,500 calories, so don't expect it to happen overnight.

If you have lost weight rapidly in the past, then

Table 3:

Area	Date	Date	Date	Date	Total lost
	1st	7th	14th	21st	
around the upper arm					
bust					
waist					

you have probably lost body fluid and not fat. The body cannot burn more than 1–2 lb (0.4–0.9 kg) of fat per week. If you imagine a 2 pint (1 litre) jelly mould, full of semi-solidified lard and coloured yellow, that is what 1 lb (0.4 kg) of fat looks like.

If you are losing 0.5–2 lb (0.2–0.9 kg) per week by following this programme, that is a clear indication that you are losing fat and not just water – which is exactly what you should be aiming for. How quickly you will see results depends on several factors, including:

1 How well you adhere to the programme (food and exercise)
2 Your dietary history, i.e. if you have lost weight and regained it several times
3 How long you have been overweight
4 Your age
5 Your sex

There is no set pattern that everyone can follow to lose the same amount of weight. If you follow this programme with a partner or friend, then you should not expect both of you to lose weight at exactly the same rate. It doesn't mean that one of you is doing 'better' than the other, it just means that your bodies are responding at a different rate, which is quite normal.

LEARNING TO BE PATIENT

Quick fix diets do not reduce the amount of fat on your body, so don't be fooled into believing the scales tell the whole story. One of the members at my club,

Tracy, has lost a staggering 14′ (36 cm) in a couple of months, but it only shows as 7 lb (3 kg) on the scales. Nevertheless, she has streamlined her figure and looks fantastic. Her new shape is down to the fact that she has lost body fat and not body fluid. She has also increased the amount of muscle tissue she has due to toning exercises, which in turn enables her to burn more calories on a daily basis.

You may find people who have used other diet programmes and lost more weight on the scales but, because they haven't actually lost body fat, don't look any better. In fact they often look more flabby than when they started, whereas Tracy has gone down a dress size and has really toned up her body and improved her shape.

When people lose weight quickly and end up looking flabby, they often put it down to 'loose skin' as a result of their weight loss. This is not true. The 'loose skin' is in fact fat, lying under the surface of the skin. There is no such thing as loose skin due to fat loss. Fat is stored under the skin and, as excess fat is lost, the skin is literally drawn in. If I think how large my tummy got during each of my three pregnancies and how toned and tight it is now, I know that could not have happened without my losing the extra fat I stored during those months. Some of that fat was stored underneath my skin, which made it flabby for the first few months after my babies were born. But I lost the extra fat and regained my figure through a programme of sensible eating and regular exercise. That's how you can lose weight and regain your figure too.

WHEN TO WEIGH

Almost everybody I have met who is overweight has been obsessed with the scales. Many people on weight loss programmes weigh themselves after every meal. This is tragic, because it does not give you any idea of how much body fat you are losing.

If you do want to weigh yourself, keep it to once a week, or ideally once a fortnight. Your body weight can fluctuate by about 1–1.5 lb (0.4–0.7 kg) on a daily basis – this is quite normal. What you must look for is a downward trend. You may even like to make a small graph and plot your progress. If the line is gradually going down over a period of time, then you are losing body fat and changing your shape. Don't worry if you have weeks where you lose little or nothing, or even gain a bit. This is quite normal. Just look at the overall trend and don't feel tied to the scales.

When you weigh yourself, you can also use this time to reflect on your progress in other areas. I have found that when people take time to review what they have eaten or how much they have exercised, it really helps them to stay on track. If you have been recording what you eat, take time to sit and look through your log and see if you can identify any areas where you could improve the balance of your food.

If you are not weighing yourself and are measuring your progress by body shape, then you will still find it beneficial to sit and reflect on what you have been doing and on your results so far. As with the scales, don't expect to be 'perfect' in every respect.

When you are doing your review, make sure you also record how many times you have exercised.

Exercise combined with changing your eating habits is the key to losing weight and changing your shape for good. Some of the exercise programmes in this book are only 10 minutes long, so no excuses like 'I haven't got time'! A combination of the right balance of food and exercise will give you the shape you want and make you feel better too. More on exercise later.

LET FOOD BE A PLEASURE

Once you get used to eating lots of carbohydrate foods and reducing meat and dairy products, you will find you can eat plenty without feeling hungry or as though you are missing out on anything. This isn't a life of deprivation! If it is your birthday or a special occasion and you want a piece of cheesecake, have it and enjoy it. As long as the overall balance of what you eat is correct, you can enjoy the occasional treat without feeling bad about it. After all, food is one of life's pleasures and should be enjoyed.

My favourite saying sums it all up: 'It's not what you do between Christmas and New Year, it's what you do between New Year and Christmas!'

Chapter 2

Body Composition

We are all different. Not only do we have individual personalities and features (thank goodness) but we all have our own individual genetic make up. Although we can see various patterns or traits that seem more common to some, we all have our very unique blue-print.

However, there are some characteristics that we all possess, characteristics that make us human. For example, we all have a skeleton, a framework that enables us to move. It also provides protection, in particular for delicate organs such as the brain and the reproductive organs. Of course the skeleton cannot move by itself, it requires muscles to pull the bones closer together to create movement.

'I AM OVERWEIGHT BECAUSE I HAVE HEAVY BONES!'

The size of your skeleton determines your height and to some extent your build, but do not kid yourself that you are overweight because you have a large frame. The bones themselves are incredibly light. They have to be, otherwise we wouldn't be able to move as freely as we can. Their centre is an almost hollow honeycomb. If your bones were solid, they would be so heavy that you would not be able to lift your arms, let alone run, walk or skip. So much for the excuse that your weight problem is due to your bones!

Just as your skeleton does not determine your weight, neither does it determine how much muscle you have. That depends almost entirely on how active you are. We all know that if you are injured and spend long periods of time confined to bed, muscle wastage occurs. If you have ever seen anyone with a broken leg that has been in plaster for some time, you will have noticed a difference between the injured leg and the good leg that has been working extra hard to support the body weight by itself. This is simply an exaggerated illustration of what is happening to all of your muscles now, if you do not exercise. The difference might just not be so noticeable over a short period of time, partly because the muscle you are losing is being replaced by body fat. In fact you may even see an increase in total size, as 1 lb (0.4 kg) of body fat takes up much more room than 1 lb of muscle.

So in order to change your shape, you need to get moving and replace body fat with muscle. But first, what shape are you in now?

WORKING OUT YOUR BODY MASS

One method of determining your body composition which is far more accurate than just going by the scales is to assess your body mass index (BMI). This is a method commonly used by scientists and researchers. It involves only two measurements and a calculation between your weight and your height. The procedure is to multiply your weight in pounds by 700, then divide the answer by your height in inches, and then divide the answer by your height in inches again. It sounds complicated, but with a calculator will only take you a few moments, and will tell you how much of your body is fat and how much is lean body mass (LBM). It is impossible to tell this from the scales, and yet it is much more relevant if you are trying to lose weight.

Here is an example of a BMI calculation:

weight in pounds = 144
height = 65′
144 x 700 = 100,800
100,800 ÷ 65 = 1,550.7692
1,550.7692 ÷ 65 = 23.85

Total BMI = 23.85

If the figure you end up with is less than 27, you are considered to be within a normal range as far as the health effects of being overweight are concerned. The threshold for being underweight is 18. Your BMI may be 26 and you may feel as though you would like to lose a little more body fat, even though you are within the recommended range for health. This is fine, as long as you do not go below 18.

It takes some time for your BMI to change, so don't expect to calculate it every week and see a drastic change. A calculation every 4–6 weeks is sufficient. Remember, you are not on a 'diet' – this is a long-term programme to change your shape.

MEN ARE DIFFERENT

There is an essential difference between men and women as far as body weight and composition are concerned: men carry more muscle and less body fat.

Unfair, but true! The reason, as I explained in detail in my first book, *Fat to Flat*, is that women are prepared by nature for child-bearing. A growing baby has to be nourished in order to develop and nature ensures that there is enough fuel to do the job by allocating women extra fat storage.

Muscles have to metabolize nutrients constantly in order to perform daily functions and remain healthy. So it is the amount of muscle tissue that determines the number of calories our body requires or burns every day. It follows therefore that men can eat more than women without gaining weight, simply because they have the potential to burn more calories on a daily basis. They also have the potential to burn more calories when they exercise because of this extra muscle. Fat, on the other hand, requires no energy. It will sit in the fat cell quite happily until it is released to provide energy.

THE NEED FOR FAT

Some people think of a 'perfect' figure as one without any fat, yet body fat is essential. We all, men and women, need to store a certain amount. It protects internal organs and insulates us, as well as providing a reserve fuel supply. This is essential for survival, as it can be converted into fuel for the brain in an emergency.

It is very difficult to change the number of fat cells on your body, as they are laid down in the womb, the first year and adolescence, although some research has shown that obese patients may be able to increase their number in some cases. There is absolutely no evidence to show or even suggest that you can reduce the number. Once they are laid down that's it, you are stuck with them. Don't despair, though – what you *can* change is the amount of fat you put into each fat cell. When they are empty they take up so little room that they do not change your body shape; they are flat, just like an empty balloon. When they are full, they become like a balloon filled with air, and although they can be relatively light when compared with muscle weight, they take up a lot of space and increase your overall size.

You must keep the genetic factor in perspective. Remember, even if you do inherit a large number of fat cells, you do not have to fill them up.

When you can't get into your jeans, don't blame it all on your genes!

APPLES AND PEARS

The pattern of fat deposition can be put in two categories:

Android obesity – This can be seen in both sexes, but is more common in males. Fat is stored mainly in the upper half of the body, around the shoulders and the nape of the neck, and above the belly button. People with this shape are often very strong and carry quite a lot of muscle. Diabetes, high blood pressure and other problems associated with being overweight are more common in this group.

Gynoid obesity – This can be seen in both sexes, but is more common in females. Fat is usually stored below the belly button, on the hips, thighs and buttocks.

People in this group suffer less from the medical problems associated with android obesity. However, they usually have less muscle tissue.

MEN AND WOMEN

The sexual differences between how and where men and women store their fat appears to start as early as five years old. Even at this early stage, fat storage is at least in part determined by how active you are, which in turn determines your rate of muscle growth and development. After the age of five, the fat mass of females is approximately double that of males of the same age.

The male pattern of fat distribution is established around puberty. It varies from that of women in that most of the fat is stored around the abdominal area. It is common for men to have a rounded belly but quite lean legs. This is due to the presence of male hormones, known as androgens, which are responsible for the number of fat cells laid down.

By the time puberty is ending, there is a noticeable difference in body shape between the sexes. Girls tend to store more fat on their lower body, around the hips, thighs and buttocks, although there are many variations on this 'pear' theme. If you think about it, it is quite logical that women store fat lower down, as this helps us to balance. If we carried this excess weight on our upper body, we would be so top heavy that we would literally fall over! If it has to go somewhere (and unfortunately it does!) then the bottom half is definitely the best place for it.

The only place where fat is thicker on men than

women is the nape of the neck. There is no logical explanation for this; however, I have no doubt that it served some useful purpose at some stage in our development.

DO WE REALLY LOSE FAT FROM THE TOP FIRST?

This is a common idea and there really does seem to be a difference in the way in which fat is metabolized from different deposits.

Research has shown that fat is released more readily into the bloodstream from the abdominal fat cells than from the lower body fat cells. So abdominal fat tends to interfere more with the heart and circulatory system and is therefore associated with a greater risk of suffering from heart disease. Women therefore have the advantage as far as the health consequences of fat storage are concerned. They are also protected from heart disease prior to menopause by female hormones. After menopause, however, this is not the case and they become as 'at risk' as men. Because of this pattern of fat release, however, many women do find that they lose weight from the top first.

Having said that, it *is* possible to lose fat from the hips and thighs, even if it is the last fat to go. One lady, Sandra, at my club in Leicestershire, has a typical pear-shaped figure. With a combination of watching her food intake and regular exercise (three times per week in the gym doing aerobic and toning work) she has lost 2 inches (5 cm) off her thighs, 2 inches from her hips and only 1 inch (2.5 cm) from her bust, and she looks great.

The only time when women do lose fat from their

thighs first is when they are breastfeeding. This makes perfect sense, as that is what the fat was stored there for in the first place. Many new mums make the mistake of thinking they will not breastfeed because it means they will not be able to diet. In fact it is the best way of losing those extra inches, quite apart from the fact that breast milk is the best possible nourishment for a baby. By not breastfeeding, you are inhibiting the mechanism that will release the most fat from your hips and thighs, and help you to regain your figure.

NO ENERGY

Although some body fat is necessary, there are many disadvantages to storing *excess* body fat, quite apart from how you look. Fat is shuttling in and out of fat cells all of the time, according to how active you are and therefore how much fat you need for fuel. It is carried in the blood and an excess amount means the heart has to work harder to pump the blood the extra distance. As a result, the heart can become stressed and overworked.

A lot of the fat we eat is also transported around in the lymphatic system, which is a network of vessels running alongside the blood vessels that carry fluids around the body. This system can easily become clogged up and sluggish if it has to transport a lot of fat. This has a knock-on effect on the immune system, which is then weakened. These problems are compounded if you do not exercise.

CHANGING YOUR SHAPE

Understanding your body type and how it functions will help you with your weight loss programme. If you understand how the body metabolizes and burns fat – and that difference isn't always noticeable on the scales at first – you will appreciate the results that you will get if you follow this programme. Remember, I cannot show you how to become taller or shorter or change your genetic inheritance, but I *can* help you to make the best of the shape you have. I can teach you and encourage you to follow a weight loss programme that means fat loss, not just weight on the scales. This is the best way to improve your body shape, to lose fat and to tone up your muscles so that you look and feel great.

WHAT SHAPE ARE YOU?

As well as apple and pear shapes, body types are often categorized under three main headings: endomorph, mesomorph and ectomorph. These categories were originally devised by a man named Sheldon. He called the process 'somatotyping'.

The characteristics of each body type are as follows:

Endomorph – This is a generally rounded shape, with soft contours of the body, very fleshy. There are often high square shoulders and a short neck. The abdomen usually protrudes.

Mesomorph – This is a squarer shape, athletic looking, with large bones and thick muscles. The arms, legs and trunk are usually thick and strong. The waist is usually slimmer than the chest. There are broad shoulders and well developed back muscles. Even the skin may appear thicker. This is the most common shape for élite athletes.

Ectomorph – This shape is long and slender, and often very lean. Bones are small and muscles thin. It is common to have drooping or rounded shoulders. The body is not necessarily tall, but the arms and legs are long in relation to the trunk. The tummy is flat and there is little curvature of the lower spine (lumbar region). Shoulders are narrow.

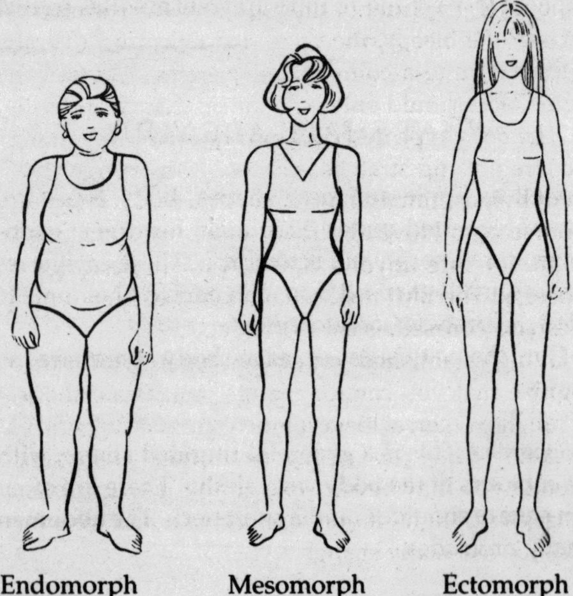

In reality, it is almost impossible to find someone who fits a particular type exactly. We are all a percentage of each. However, you can see characteristics of a particular type in certain people. For example the Princess of Wales is mainly ectomorph, although she also has some mesomorph qualities.

Look at the diagrams of the three main body types and see which most represents your own body shape. Don't expect to be a perfect match – it is just to give you an idea.

A more complicated method of assessing your body type was also developed by Sheldon, using detailed body measurements taken from the triceps (the muscle at the back of your arm), the back of the shoulder, the front of the hips, the calf, the elbow, the knee, the biceps, the overall weight and overall height. It's quite a complicated process, as you can imagine, and should only be done by trained individuals. The body type descriptions range from 'Walking sticks, fragile and stretched out' to 'Rhinoceros, sturdiest of living animals, built to resist armoured tanks'! Of course we all love to put ourselves into categories, but I'm not sure anyone would want to be called a rhinoceros! The BMI method explained earlier, which you can do yourself, is far more practical.

Having established your body type, you need to recognize that you cannot change your basic shape. You can, however, achieve a much slimmer version of the same shape by eating well and exercising. Although you may be an apple or a pear shape when you are overweight, if you lose body fat and tone up, that shape can really change.

SPOT REDUCTION – THE MYTH

The programmes in this book will enable you to lose fat from all of your fat cells. You cannot 'spot reduce', i.e. lose fat from just some of them. Spot reduction is probably the biggest myth surrounding the weight loss industry. It is physiologically impossible to burn fat from your thighs, for example, with one exercise and from your tummy with another. What you *can* do is to lose excess fat from all of your fat cells and tone up the muscles in one particular area to give you a much firmer shape.

It makes sense that if you store most of your fat around your tummy and you then diet and exercise, that is where you will see the most difference. If you had large stores of fat on your earlobe and you were to exercise regularly on a rowing machine, you would burn the fat from your earlobe, although you did not use your ears to do the exercise!

Researchers used tennis players to prove the point. Surely if you could burn fat from one particular area, then a sport such as tennis, where one arm is used far more than the other, would clearly show that right-handed players have less fat on their right arm than on their left. The study showed quite clearly that in *every* case the amount of fat stored around the right arm was exactly the same as that stored around the left, even though the muscles on the right arm were sometimes more developed.

THE NEW YOU

So, if you have a particular area of your body which you want to change, you need a programme which will burn fat overall. You can then exercise the particular area you want to work on to improve the muscle tone there, which will give you a better shape. For example, if you want to lose fat from your buttocks, follow the nutritional advice and the recipes in this book and do regular aerobic exercise to train your body to burn more fat, followed by the toning exercises designed specifically for that area. As the fat starts to come off, your buttocks will become firmer and tighter, and your shape will begin to change.

An important point to remember is that both diet and exercise are necessary. If you use diet alone, then you are unlikely to succeed. If you are lucky, you could reduce the amount of fat you store, but without exercises to tone up the muscles, although you may end up with a slightly smaller bottom, it will be just as flabby. Then in a very short space of time you will probably regain the weight, and more besides. If you follow this programme, however, you will end up much slimmer and firmer – whatever shape you are!

Chapter 3

Metabolism – Teach your Body to Burn More Fat

We often hear the word 'metabolism' – but do we really know what it means? Like so many other 'technical' words it is often bandied about by manufacturers who claim their latest product 'speeds it up'. But would that help to change your shape?

'Metabolism' actually refers to the synthesis or combining of all the reactions that occur in the body. If you know something about these processes, it will help you to understand just what impact your food and your activity levels can have on the amount of calories you are able to burn, and this will help you to tell fact from fiction when the next 'metabolism booster' product comes along.

We can simplify metabolism a little by breaking it down into two main categories:

Anabolism. This is the building or putting together of molecules. The general process of growth and repair that goes on continuously in the body depends on it. Anabolism is a process which requires energy (from food) in order to join small molecules together to form larger molecules. It takes place within all of our cells, and enables them to divide and form new cells. The cells themselves also have to maintain their own structure via the process of anabolism. Everyday functions such as producing hormones also come under this classification.

The easy way to remember that anabolism means building up is to think of anabolic steroids, which are drugs taken to help build muscle tissue. People who take anabolic steroids literally want to build up their size. Unfortunately, this can lead to health problems in the long term and is not to be recommended.

Catabolism. This means breaking down or decomposing molecules; it is the opposite of anabolism. Larger molecules are broken down to form smaller molecules. This includes the breakdown of food molecules in the intestine and ultimately within the cells. It also includes the breaking down of fat molecules from their storage sites (adipose tissue) as well as the breakdown of micro-organisms in certain blood cells that protect us from infection. Catabolism releases energy.

AEROBIC AND ANAEROBIC EXERCISE

Catabolism of fat depends on several factors. First, the presence of oxygen, which means the body has to be functioning 'aerobically'. This means that the heart has to be able to pump oxygen around the body to the working muscles at a fast enough rate to provide a constant supply of oxygen to the small structures within the muscles, where the actual breakdown of the fat occurs. These structures are called mitochondrion. They are small capsules that contain oxygen, small carbohydrate molecules that are broken down to form glucose, or blood sugar, and small fat molecules, or fatty acids. Together these three elements can be broken down to produce energy, or a force that will enable the muscle to contract or move.

Examples of aerobic activity vary for individuals, depending on fitness levels, but generally include brisk walking, light jogging, swimming, cycling,rowing, etc. Of course for one person a brisk walk might seem very easy and therefore probably wouldn't be enough to significantly increase the amount of fat being burnt. But for someone who does not exercise at all, a brisk walk can seem like a real effort and can actually take them above their aerobic capability, which means that their heart is not strong enough to pump the blood carrying oxygen to the working muscles as fast as it is being used up. Therefore they end up with a deficit and begin to work anaerobically, which means 'without oxygen'.

The anaerobic method of energy production *does not* use fat. Carbohydrate is burnt in the form of glucose without oxygen and without fat. When you work anaerobically, the amount of time you can continue is very limited, partly because the supplies of glycogen (small molecules of glucose in the muscles) are limited and therefore run out very quickly and partly because you're not using oxygen. Anaerobic exercise is usually high intensity exercise – sprinting, for example.

Think of the fat in the mitochondrion like coal: it has to have oxygen in order to burn. If there is little or no oxygen, the fire goes out. The more oxygen there is, on the other hand, the faster the coal can burn. If we liken the fat in the mitochondrion to coal, the principle is exactly the same.

We all have an aerobic capability, which is dependent on our fitness level, i.e. the strength of our heart muscle, which ultimately determines how much blood gets pumped around the body. This aerobic range can be quite varied. Of course, you are breathing as you are reading this (hopefully!) therefore at the moment you are working aerobically and in the process you are burning or metabolizing a small amount of fat along with some glycogen. If you were to start walking around, the amount of fat you are burning would increase slightly. This system, however, is quite slow, which means that you can't just jump up, walk around briskly for 10 minutes and burn fat. Unfortunately it can take several minutes to actually get the process going.

Let's think again about the fire. When you build a fire, you need to use paper or small twigs that burn quickly in order to get it going, as the coal takes much longer to start to burn. Of course once it does start to burn, it lasts much longer than the paper or twigs, which would have long since burnt out. In the same way your body burns glycogen first of all, but there isn't enough glycogen to keep the fire going without something longer lasting. So after a time (usually several minutes, depending on how hard you are working), it starts to burn fat, which is long lasting and produces lots of energy. Providing the level you are exercising at is low to moderate, you can keep going for longer. This means improved stamina, which will help make you feel fitter and cope with everyday tasks more easily. You are also burning fat.

Unfortunately, we cannot burn fat without glycogen. The whole complicated process of catabolism which breaks down fat to provide energy is dependent on both oxygen and carbohydrate being present. If that were not the case, every time we wanted to lose weight, we could just stop eating for a while, do lots of exercise until we had used up all the excess fat and then start eating again. No wonder it sounds too good to be true – it is!

So what can we learn from this process of catabolism that will help us to burn fat more effectively? First, it is clear that we *must* exercise in order to burn more fat. Although we are burning fat all the time, the amount is quite small in relation to the amount we can store. In fact we have the potential to store billions of calories as fat, but an average person will store only about 1,500 calories of carbohydrate (in the form of glycogen). If you exercise regularly, you are more likely to burn more calories than you consume and the deficit will be met by taking fat from the fat cells. If you eat more calories than you use, you will continue to increase the amount of fat you store. It is quite a simple equation!

APPETITE – OR FOOD ON DEMAND?

Although individual metabolic rates do vary, in my experience most people are overweight because they overeat. The body has a demand for food of course, which must be met in order for life to continue. But what makes us overeat?

How often do you hear someone say, 'Oh, I can't help the amount I eat. I have a large appetite'? I was flicking through my thesaurus to find another word that could be used instead and was amazed at the amount of alternatives I found. Would you associate 'appetite' with 'longing', 'need', 'demand', 'desire', 'require', 'yearn', 'expect', 'crave' and even 'lust'?! It makes you think, doesn't it? Just what do we mean when we say we are hungry? I doubt that anyone reading this book has ever been really hungry. Of course you may have skipped a meal or not eaten as much as you would have liked, but hungry in the true sense of the word?

TRUE OR FALSE APPETITE

Have you ever enjoyed a really nice meal and been totally satisfied, only to be offered an hour or two later a cup of tea and a scone or some tasty savoury? How many times have you eaten because you thought, 'Oh yes, I am starting to get a little peckish, I just about have room for that'? Then, once you get the taste for it, you manage to squeeze in room for another one (or two!)

We are constantly eating when we are not hungry. Not only do we eat when we don't need to, but we often eat when our digestive system is positively overburdened and doesn't want any more food.

As mentioned earlier, eating calorie-laden food may not be enough to satisfy your hunger, if you are not supplying the body with all the nutrients it requires. Even though you are eating far more calories than you need, the body will feel 'hungry' for food that contains nutrients. If you answer this hunger with more calorie-rich foods which do not contain nutrients, then the cycle will go on and on, you will gain more and more weight and become more and more lethargic – sound familiar? Are you always hungry? If so, perhaps your body is trying to tell you it needs more nutrients.

Alternatively, some food intolerances may cause

fluid retention or cravings for certain foods, particularly sweet-tasting foods.

The sense by which hunger is produced is a complicated one and there are several different theories. Most experts do agree, however, that it is the nervous system that ultimately brings about the sensation of hunger, when stimulated by a part of the brain called the hypothalamus. The endocrine system is also linked to this process.

Hunger is a perfectly normal sensation. It creates a desire for food that is quite pleasant. Sometimes you experience a pleasant sensation in the mouth, a desire rather than a craving or desperate need. If you have a false appetite, you are more likely to experience unpleasant sensations, even an irritation.

We often mistake other sensations for that of hunger. True hunger just demands food, not a specific kind of food or a specific product – just any food. It is satisfied with plain fare. It does not require luxurious dishes. The compulsive eater, who is not genuinely hungry, quite often wants or craves something to eat that is specifically sweet or savoury. They 'fancy' a certain kind of food. The more they think about this kind of food, the more they want it. Their mouth begins to water and they tell themselves, wrongly, that they are hungry. They need something to satisfy their taste buds, not their hunger. I know this because I have done it myself. At one time I could devour two or three chocolate bars without a second glance. It would only take a picture or an image and my taste buds were screaming out for a chocolate fix.

How often have you been sitting at the theatre or at the cinema, quite happy and contented, until the interval, when the usherette appears in front of you with a tray full of goodies, sweets, ice cream and fizzy drinks? You go from not wanting anything to a sudden lust for something, made worse by the sight or smells of all those other people tucking in. It is very unlikely that you were hungry at all, but something visual or an aroma stimulated your taste buds and you eat or drank food that your body didn't want and certainly didn't need!

Chances are these will be the excess calories that you consume more often than you probably realize. These are probably the calories that cause you to gain weight. Have you ever heard the slogan 'Just Say No!'? Well, if your taste buds are telling you they want something, just say no.

BE AWARE

We should all listen to our bodies more often. We regularly eat because it is 'time to eat', perhaps lunchtime or the time you have your evening meal. Do you ever really listen to your body or do you just go along with the normal routine, often dictated by social events or other people, eating when you do not need to and when your digestive system really needs to be at rest?

Even when someone is ill, there is a constant desire to give them something to eat. It is seen almost as a sign of recovery. 'He looked much better today. I managed to get some soup down him.' The poor patient hardly has a say in the matter! The fact is, when we are ill, our digestive system needs to slow down, so that some of the valuable energy it takes to digest food can be used to heal our body instead.

If you do eat when you are ill, it often results in

sickness or diarrhoea, as the body cannot cope with food at this time. We expel the food because it is a burden on the digestive system and we have to get rid of it. This often slows down the recovery time. Of course, I am not suggesting you should fast completely when you are ill, but listen to your body. If you don't feel a genuine need for food, don't eat. Just make sure you drink lots of fresh water.

You must learn your limitations in food consumption. If you respect these, you will not only lose weight, but you will be more likely to enjoy good health. If you continue to overeat, you will not only gain weight, but you are more likely to become ill and suffer disease. You will find that your TLC programme will help you learn how to control what and how much you eat.

Now let's look at food in greater detail.

Part 2: So Just What Should You Eat?

Chapter 4

Food Groups

We need food to nourish our bodies, to give us energy to survive, to fight infection and disease and to enable us to live life to the full. There has been a lot of media coverage over the past couple of years on 'choosing the healthy options', but often valid information is misquoted by ruthless manufacturers and advertising agencies to trick us into thinking a particular product is good for us. So just what should you eat?

Food can be divided into three main categories: fat, carbohydrate and protein. Each has a specific function in the body and provides a different range of nutrients which the body can use. Ideally, we should eat a mixture of all three, with most of our food coming from carbohydrate sources, some from fats and the smallest amount from protein. This chapter will look at carbohydrate and protein; fats are discussed in the next chapter.

CARBOHYDRATE

Why do we need so much carbohydrate and what is it exactly? Carbohydrate is very important, because it provides us with lots of vitamins and minerals. Carbohydrates can be defined as foods that have never been born, that is, they are organic. For example, an apple has never been born, nor have rice or potatoes, they come from the ground, from a seed that has grown.

Carbohydrates get their energy to grow from the sun. They convert sunlight, carbon dioxide and water into energy via a process called photosynthesis. They store the valuable nutrients they themselves need as glucose, or simple sugars. Maltose and fructose are also stored in this way. When we eat the plants, we are eating these nutrients. We are effectively interrupting the plants' own food chain in order to satisfy our own requirements.

We use the glucose from carbohydrates to provide fuel for energy. We burn it when we need to move very quickly, as it can supply immediate power, and also use it as a long-term energy supply in combination with fat.

Carbohydrates are not only important for this reason, but they also contain valuable nutrients which enable the internal organs and the nervous system to function. Carbohydrates are also needed to supply the nutrients that regulate protein and fat metabolism.

Carbohydrates are named or classified according to their structure.

SIMPLE CARBOHYDRATES, OR SUGARS

Monosaccharides (single sugars) include glucose, fructose and galactose. Fructose is found in most fruits and fruit juices, and also honey and some vegetables. It is sweeter than cane sugar and has to be modified in the liver before absorption takes place.

Disaccharides (double sugars) include lactose, which is often called 'milk sugar'; maltose, from cereal grains; and sucrose, which is found in foods such as sugar cane and sugar beet. Sucrose is composed of one molecule of fructose and one molecule of glucose and is very sweet.

Sugars are the enemy in terms of staying healthy and trying to lose weight. Too much sugar is converted to and stored as fat. And if you eat a combination of fat and sugar together, it is a one-way ticket to the fat cell – on a fast train! You should remember that next time you are tempted by a low-fat label – if the product is high in sugar, it will be converted to fat anyway!

Table sugar, a crystallized form of sucrose, is greatly overused – not only as we sprinkle it over our food and drinks, but also in the preparation of many foods such as baked beans, sweetcorn and even some soups! Salad dressings and sauces can also contain large amounts of sugar.

Sugar addiction is common and is responsible for a wide variety of health problems, from obesity to rotten teeth. It generally takes about 4–6 weeks of not having products containing lots of sugar, such as confectionery and sweet drinks, to lose the craving. Once you have got over this period, you will find that your taste buds become more sensitive to other wonderful flavours that have been previously masked by the sugar.

I have helped many people who have complained of the following symptoms:

mood swings
erratic sleep patterns
restlessness
food cravings, particularly for something sweet
headaches

Once they have removed sugar from their diet, their symptoms fade and disappear.

Another good reason for avoiding sugar is that the body can quickly and efficiently turn it into fatty acids. And, like anything else that we eat too much of, excess sugar is stored as body fat. If you constantly bombard your body with refined carbohydrates in the form of sugars, you will be adding to your fat stores, even though you are not actually eating fat, as the calorific value of the food will be high. Sugar is in effect an empty calorie.

Blood Sugar – Highs and Lows

Refined sugars, such as those that are used in many of the processed foods we eat, are digested very quickly and therefore released into our bloodstream very fast. The body cannot cope with these rapid changes, as its level of glucose needs to remain quite constant. Blood glucose levels are monitored by the hormone insulin. When they are too high, a condition known as hyperglycaemia, insulin is released from the pancreas and rapidly deals with the problem by converting the excess sugar into fat and depositing the fat molecules into our fat cells.

Unfortunately, this process is almost too efficient, as insulin not only mops up the excess, but also takes out so much glucose that we are left with low blood sugar levels. Symptoms of low blood glucose levels, or hypoglycaemia, are weakness, fatigue, insomnia, dizziness, tearfulness and even loss of consciousness. When levels are low, our adrenal glands are alerted and subsequently mobilize the body's stores of glycogen to make up the deficit.

If you eat a diet high in refined carbohydrates, you are constantly overworking your pancreas and your adrenal glands, as they have to cope with the repeated sugar rush. If your pancreas becomes so overworked that it weakens, it is not able to produce sufficient amounts of insulin. Therefore blood glucose levels remain constantly high and can be detected in the urine.

Stress, Blood Sugar and Cravings

If your adrenal glands are overworked and not able to function properly, your ability to deal with stress will be drastically reduced. Also, the delicate balance by which all of our organs and systems function together will be disrupted and disease will almost certainly occur. Many people who suffer from stress would feel much better if they simply reduced or eliminated refined sugar from their diet.

If the adrenal glands are unable to raise the blood glucose level sufficiently after the mopping up operation, then you will remain in a state of hypoglycaemia. This will cause a craving for something sweet. If you respond to this craving by having some confectionery, which contains refined sugar, although you will experience a very temporary relief, you are ultimately making the problem worse.

If you think you may be suffering from a see-saw

of high and low blood sugar, then you must cut out products containing refined sugar. But remember, this isn't a 'diet of deprivation'! Just replace them with something else. Try nibbling on raw vegetables or fruit. These foods have to be broken down gradually and digested fully before they can be released into your bloodstream, so they do not imbalance the blood sugar levels. If possible, try not to eat between meals, until the sugar cravings are under control. This may be hard if you are a regular sweet addict, but I assure you, after a few weeks you really will lose the craving.

You may find that you can satisfy a sweet craving with a piece of fruit. Fruit sugar is better than refined sugar because it has to go to the liver to be metabolized before it can enter the bloodstream, therefore the rise in blood glucose is not so rapid. One of my favourite nibbles is to dip a whole baby sweetcorn into some yoghurt or just crunch it on its own – delicious!

Most foods we eat contain the nutrients our body requires to break them down and digest them. Refined sugar contains no nutrients, so it has to draw on our reserves of nutrients supplied by other foods in order to be digested. These valuable nutrients (B_1, zinc, B_3 and chromium) could be put to far better use than metabolizing sugar, on more urgent tasks like growth and cell repair.

Although your body can turn sugar into fat, it cannot turn fat back into sugar. The fat, once stored, will only be released to be burnt as fuel during activity.

I could probably write a whole book on the reasons for avoiding refined sugar; however, I hope this gives you an insight into just a few of the problems it can cause. If you want to lose weight, then you must reduce the sugar content of your diet. Try and think of sugar as a hidden fat – as that is what it becomes in your body if you have too much.

STARCH

Apart from sugars, carbohydrates also contain starches. These are also called polysaccharides, or complex carbohydrates. They are not as simple in their structure as sugars and therefore take the body longer to break down. This is much better as it means there is a slower release of glucose into the blood. The body breaks down starch by using enzymes in the digestive system to take it apart bit by bit. An enzyme is something that either breaks down or builds up molecules. Starch itself contains not only the nutrients required to break it down, but also other valuable nutrients that the body can use for other things.

Complex carbohydrates should be the single most important aspect of your diet. If you go back several years, before refined foods became so freely available and popular, the average diet consisted of a lot of starchy foods, such as potatoes, root vegetables and whole grains such as wheat, barley and oats, and some rice and corn. In addition, the use of pesticides was not as widespread and before 1940 many more people were eating organic produce. This was a much healthier diet than the average Western one today.

You will find it much easier to lose weight if the bulk of your diet comes from complex carbohydrates. In fact, if you adopted this approach, it would be quite difficult to gain weight even if you wanted to!

Just imagine how much broccoli you would have to eat to get the same amount of calories contained in a typical chocolate bar – you couldn't do it.

If you do nothing else but increase the amount of vegetables you eat, you will be providing your body with valuable extra nutrients, i.e. vitamins, minerals, essential fatty acids and other compounds which will help you fight against disease, as well as to lose weight and change shape.

FIBRE

Complex carbohydrate foods are high in fibre. Fibre does not provide energy, but it does aid the body's process of elimination. This is because it is indigestible, so it passes through the body relatively unchanged, and promotes the churning and pushing action of the intestines. This process is called peristalsis. It enables our body to process and eliminate foods without blockage or stoppages along the way. In other words, it keeps everything moving. This is important as a backlog of food can cause toxins to be released into the body instead of eliminated. Fibre also helps to mop up excess cholesterol for excretion.

If your diet contains adequate fibre, you should be going to the toilet once or twice a day and your stools should float. If you are not this regular then you may have a problem with digestion. If this is the case it may be quite difficult for you to lose weight until you manage to get your bowels to open regularly. If your diet is low in fibre you are likely to suffer from constipation, gastrointestinal disorders and even to increase your risk of suffering from colon cancer.

Including more complex carbohydrates in the diet

will ease the problem. I would not necessarily recommend eating vast amounts of brown bread, however, because it may be that you have irritable bowel syndrome (IBS). If so, bread may make the situation worse. Some people find that when they change to a diet high in vegetables and lower in meat, they start to get wind and flatulence. This may also be due to IBS. Once you have eliminated the food that is causing the problem, the symptoms will reduce and eventually stop altogether. More on this later.

Fibre absorbs water, so when you eat a meal which is high in fibre you experience a sense of fullness, even though you haven't necessarily consumed many calories. (Fibre is almost calorie free.) So it is excellent as part of a weight loss programme.

Some people who are trying to increase the amount of fibre in their diet add bran to cereals, etc. This can pose a problem, as high levels of wheat bran can reduce the absorption of certain minerals (e.g. zinc and magnesium, which are essential for normal metabolism). If you are eating a diet which is high in refined carbohydrates, e.g. sugar, and low in complex carbohydrates, the chances are that you may well be deficient in some nutrients anyway. If you add too much bran to this equation and reduce the absorption of even more, you can end up with a diet very low in nutrients. If, on the other hand, you consume more vegetables and fruit, you are not only likely to speed up the passage of your food, but will also be increasing the amount of nutrients you consume. It is not difficult to see which is the best option.

IRRITABLE BOWEL SYNDROME (IBS)

If you are wondering why I have included a section on IBS in a weight loss book, the answer is quite simple – if you are suffering from IBS it is unlikely that you are going to be able to lose weight effectively until you have cured it. Although IBS doesn't make you fat, it does mean that your digestive process is not functioning 100 per cent and you are probably retaining fluid and storing toxins that may interfere with digestion.

Typical symptoms of IBS are frequent bloating or swelling of the abdomen, particularly after eating, together with a tendency to be constipated or to have diarrhoea. Often there is flatulence and discomfort in the bowel. It is usually caused by an intolerance to something you eat a lot of. Wheat is the most common cause in the UK, followed by dairy produce, while in America corn is the most common allergen, because it is what they eat most of.

The solution is quite simple – whatever the problem substance is, don't eat it. Of course in reality this can mean quite a change – for example, if wheat is the problem you will need to avoid bread or pasta. I had IBS for two years and after several trips to the doctor's I was told to eat more brown bread. This was the worst advice I could have been given, as it aggravated the problem. I was experiencing stomach cramps and severe bloating. A friend even asked me whether I was pregnant! When I began to study nutritional therapy, I realized what the problem was straightaway. I stopped having bread and pasta and within two or three weeks I was much better. Now I can tolerate small amounts of wheat, for example if I am out and there is only a sandwich or pasta on the menu I will have it and be OK, but if I have it too often the IBS comes straight back. Many people only have to eliminate foods for a few months to allow the bowel to heal and can then reintroduce them gradually.

If you have an intolerance such as this, it is also likely that you are retaining too much fluid and will therefore find it difficult to lose weight. I have helped many people to lose weight just by getting them to avoid wheat. Of course, wheat isn't the only culprit, and if you avoid it for several weeks and still have a problem, I suggest you see a nutritional consultant who will be able to advise you on an individual basis.

KEEPING THINGS MOVING

If you think you have some other problem with elimination, then you will find the recipes in this book contain enough fibre to get things moving. If you are using your own recipes, then you should reduce the amount of meat you use and substitute it with lots of extra vegetables. For example, if you are making a dish with mince, such as shepherd's pie or spaghetti bolognese, you can use mashed carrot and swede, which mixes in really well with the meat, tastes delicious and will make the meal much higher in carbohydrates and fibre. I use a half to a third less meat if I am using mashed vegetables such as carrot and swede. You can also use any mashed root vegetables for this process, according to your taste. Try and cook the vegetables in a minimum amount of water and use the water to make a stock or to liquidize the vegetable mixture. Don't worry if it seems a little soggy – some of the water will evaporate as you cook it. Parsnips are great cooked and mashed with potatoes.

SNEAKING THE VEGETABLES IN...

Why is it that for some people 'vegetables' is a dirty word? Children in particular screw their noses up in disgust. How can you not like something that can vary so widely in taste, texture and colour? I think it is because of school dinners. I can remember lukewarm cabbage, still dripping in water, which inevitably ran into the mashed potatoes, which were also cold and somewhat lumpy. Yuck – no wonder I didn't eat cabbage for years!

I don't believe that anyone can not like some kind of vegetable, given that there are so many to choose from and so many different ways to cook them. I don't like cooked spinach all that much, for example, but used to eat it because I knew it was good for me, then I discovered raw spinach, which tastes completely different. It is lovely in a salad, far tastier than lettuce, and eating it raw means I get more of the nutrients too – which can't be bad.

If, like me, you have children or anyone else you cook for who doesn't like veg., mashing some in with potatoes and stews, etc., is a great way to get them in without anyone noticing! You should also try mixed beans. If I am short of time I take the lazy option and buy a tin of mixed beans in spicy sauce and put them into whatever I am making. I also use red lentils, as already mentioned. This way, with luck, people won't even know they are eating the dreaded vegetables and the balance of the whole meal is changed for the good.

PROTEIN

A fact that most people find surprising is that we need less dietary protein than we do carbohydrate or fat. Nevertheless, it is true and is an important factor to consider when planning your shape-changing programme. High-protein diets can be very hazardous to your health.

WHY WE NEED PROTEIN

Protein provides us with the building materials we need to repair and form new tissues, not just for muscles, but also for blood, skin, hair, nails and internal organs, including the heart and the brain. We also need protein to help us form hormones, which control many body functions, including growth, sexual development and metabolism. Protein helps to maintain the correct level of acidity in the blood and tissues and regulates water balance. The enzymes that our body uses to build up or break down food molecules are also made from protein. Another of its important functions is helping our immune system to build antibodies to fight infection. The cells that carry oxygen around in our blood, haemoglobin, are also made essentially from protein. So you can see it has many functions and this makes it even more surprising that we need so little of it.

TOO MUCH PROTEIN

Protein should make up no more than 15 per cent of our total daily dietary intake. Many people greatly exceed that ratio and therefore regularly supply their body with excess protein calories which are converted and stored as fat. Even body-builders need very little protein. It is a mistake to think that if you want to build muscle you should have raw eggs for breakfast and a whole chicken for lunch! Anyone following this kind of regime is certainly consuming far too much protein. As a result the delicate balance in the body between acid and alkaline is disrupted and many digestive problems can occur. It also means that the diet is very high in fat, in particular saturated fat, which leads to numerous health problems.

If you are eating a high-protein diet which is low in complex carbohydrate, then you are giving your body too much of something that it does not need and not enough of the vital nutrients that it does need.

AMINO ACIDS

Our body breaks protein down into tiny molecules called amino acids. Think of these amino acids as lego bricks. The body takes in protein made up of lots of lego bricks, breaks it down into single bricks, absorbs these bricks and then reconstructs them into a shape that is usable. However it can only do this if the diet is supplying all the ingredients and tools for the job. And there are some essential amino acids that our body cannot make. As these are essential to health, we must include them in our diet.

If you eat meat, you are in effect eating amino acids that have already been processed by the animal into proteins. These are called 'complete proteins' as they contain all the essential amino acids you require. If you are a vegetarian, you need to do the converting in your own body. This means you have to eat a mixture of proteins from different sources, such as vegetables, nuts, seeds and wholegrain cereals in order to have all the ingredients required to do the job. That way you take in all the essential amino acids that your body requires. If you eat a wide range of vegetables, pulses and wholegrains, then you do not have to worry, you will automatically be getting everything you need.

It is a mistake to think of meat as the primary source of protein when there are so many other excellent foods that contain not only all the protein you require, but also many other nutrients, without the saturated fat that is inevitably found in meat. If you consume complex carbohydrates in the form of vegetables, some seeds and wholegrains, you will already be meeting your body's requirement for protein.

HIGH-PROTEIN WEIGHT LOSS DIETS

Many people have achieved short-term weight loss on a high-protein diet. This is because the fat contained in high-protein foods gives a feeling of fullness that can last a long time. The reason for this is that the rate at which fats are digested is slow and our stomach doesn't want any more food until it has processed what it already contains.

If we eat large amounts of protein, though, we

produce more ammonia. The body has to convert this into urea which we can expel, but before this process is complete the ammonia can cause damage to the liver, kidneys and even the brain. High-protein diets also increase your chances of developing allergies or food intolerances, as the digestive system is constantly overloaded. They have been linked to osteoporosis, a condition in which the strength of the bones is lost as they begin to break down inside and crumble. Too much protein causes the body to 'dump' vital calcium, which cannot then be used to build or strengthen the bones.

Also, if you are eating a diet high in protein, you are probably not eating enough carbohydrate, because the high-protein diets are very filling. If you reduce the amount of carbohydrate that you eat, then you are reducing your body's natural ability to store vital fluid. A single gram (0.03 oz) of carbohydrate enables the body to store 3 grams (0.1 oz) of fluid, therefore for every gram of carbohydrate that you reduce from your diet, you are also losing 3 grams of water. This is not excess water, it is fluid that our cells desperately need in order to function. All of the reactions that take place in our body take place in a fluid or 'wet' environment. Even energy is produced in body fluids. So, if you reduce the amount of fluid you should normally retain, you can cause serious problems for the body's many different systems.

Losing body fluid can have quite a drastic effect on your weight, even though you have not lost any body fat. I recently met a lady who had lost 2 stone (13 kg) on a high-protein diet. She had been eating lots of meat, very few vegetables and no fruit, and had done no exercise. Despite the weight loss, she looked awful. Her skin was so loose and flabby, it literally hung from under her arms. She was unable to wear a short-sleeved dress because it looked so bad and would only wear trousers because her legs were so flabby. Her skin was very grey, she said she had little energy and felt very 'bunged up'. That was because she *was* bunged up; she was full of the saturated fat in the meat and lacked the vital nutrients supplied by vegetables and fruit. She was also showing signs of being dehydrated, such as mood swings, heavy-leggedness and headaches. No wonder she looked and felt awful.

Don't worry – by following the TLC programme, you can tone up, lose weight and change shape without these problems!

Chapter 5
What is Fat?

Fat, like vegetables, is a dirty word for some. The topic can be a very complex one and it is true that some fats really are harmful to our health, but others are vital. It's not just the fats we buy but also how we store and prepare them that determines whether or not they are helpful or detrimental to our health.

I am always very concerned about the amount of 'fat phobia' around. In fact most of us have probably suffered from it at some point in recent years and have tried to reduce the amount of fat in our diet. It is certainly true that many of us eat too much fat, or more specifically too much saturated fat, but did you know that you can eat a high-fat diet and still be deficient in the essential fats your body needs? Many of the 'good' fats or oils we need to eat get lumped together with the fats and oils that we do not need and by trying to avoid fat in the diet, we can easily deprive our body of vital nutrients that we need to survive.

Unfortunately, we use the same word for fat on the body and fat in the diet. This can be very confusing! In this section I will talk about fat on the body *(see also Chapter 2)* and then move on to the more complicated subject of fat in the diet.

YOUR BODY NEEDS FAT

Body fat has a bad reputation. This is quite unfair, as it is not only preferable to have adequate supplies of body fat, but it is essential to maintain health and even life. We may not like it, but we need fat on and in our body for several reasons:

1 As fuel storage in case of famine
2 For insulation and warmth
3 For the protection of delicate organs
4 As a transport system for immune cells

Fats in the form of lipids are an integral part of cell membranes, so we are utterly dependent on some forms of fat to maintain our normal healthy structure. Fats are also needed to absorb the fat-soluble vitamins A, D, E and K – after all, if they are fat soluble, there has to be some fat for them to be soluble in! Fat also aids vitamin D absorption. This in turn helps the process of absorbing calcium.

The percentage of fat on the average body varies enormously and is determined by a) genetics; b) what you eat; and c) how much or how little exercise you do. There is, however, a natural range for the amount of fat that we should 'ideally' carry: between 15 and 28 per cent. This figure varies for men and women. The amount of fat that women carry typically falls between 20 and 30 per cent, if they are quite slim. Men naturally carry approximately 10 per cent less. A lean man may have about 15 per cent body fat, which would be very low for a woman. In fact if women do reduce their body fat to this level, it is common for them to stop menstruating. This can lead to many serious health problems, including osteoporosis. Of course, in reality, a woman who exercises her muscles can be stronger than a man who is completely inactive and has very poor muscle tone. So men are *potentially* stronger.

Why do women store 10 per cent more fat than men? As already mentioned, the fact is that nature gave women more plentiful supplies of fat to feed a growing baby. Unfortunately we keep these extra stores whether we have a baby to feed or not!

FAT STORES

So why do we store our potential energy as fat? The answer is of course that nature knows best! Fat is simply the best method of fuel storage available. It can be packaged up into tiny little cells and tucked away for us to use as and when we need it. Most cells in the body are composed of 70 per cent water, but a fat cell is made up mainly of fat.

Each gram of fat we store contains more than twice as many calories (or potential energy) as carbohydrate, which we can only store in very limited amounts as glycogen. Whereas the fat we eat goes through very few changes in order to be converted into body fat, carbohydrate has to be broken down into glycogen. A lot of this work is done in the liver, which is constantly synthesizing carbohydrate into glucose molecules which can be transported in the blood to the working muscles or body tissues. The capacity for the muscles to store extra glucose is very limited and once their stores have run out they have to wait for the next 'batch' from the liver. From this we can begin to see what an important role the liver plays in metabolism and losing or gaining weight.

LOSING FAT

Although we need a certain amount of body fat, recent research has shown that people carrying excess amounts are at higher risk of suffering from many diseases, including coronary heart disease (CHD) and cancer.

As already mentioned, in order to decrease the amount of body fat we must replace the high-calorie, fat- and sugar-laden foods we commonly eat with nutrient rich wholefoods, such as fruit, vegetables, wholegrain cereals and seeds. Then not only will we lose the excess fat, but we will also feel better, have more energy and an improved skin, and we are more likely to slow down the degenerative or ageing process.

In real terms, as already explained, this doesn't necessarily mean changing what you eat completely, but it does mean changing the proportions. For example, if you eat meals that consist primarily of meat, with just a few vegetables, then you have got the balance all wrong. If you want to lose weight and improve your health, the majority of what you eat must come from carbohydrate, or plant based, foods.

However lean a cut of meat looks, it is literally saturated with fat. The animals that we eat store fat within their muscles to provide them with energy. Just think, it isn't really *your* fat that makes you fat, but the fat of the animal you're eating! Don't think that just because you take the skin off your chicken or trim off the excess visible fat that it has all gone – far from it. The fat has solidified within the muscle and it will solidify within your muscles too, once you have eaten it. And what you cannot store in the fat cells within your muscles will be stored in other fat cells around your body and under your skin.

MUSCLES BURN FAT

Without doubt, the best way to lose fat is to increase the amount of muscle or muscle tone. As already explained, fat is metabolized, or burnt, in the mitochondrion, which are small structures within the muscle. There is no other place in the body where we can burn fat. If you exercise your muscles aerobically, then the number of mitochondrion in the muscle increases, which means a direct increase in the body's ability to burn fat *(see pages 108 and 119 for more information on choosing your exercise programme)*. On the other hand, if you don't exercise, then the muscles literally shrink and their ability to burn fat is reduced.

Muscles naturally shrink anyway as we get older (the process is called 'atrophy') and it is common for the percentage of body fat to increase, but if you do not exercise the shrinkage is accelerated. Atrophy can be reversed, however, and lost muscle tissue replaced; this process is called 'hypertrophy'.

Less muscle tissue means you need fewer calories on a daily basis. If you continue to eat the same amount, it then has the same effect as eating more, i.e. you store the excess calories you are now unable to burn as fat.

If you took two people who weighed the same, but one exercised and had a higher percentage of muscle – let's call him Fred – and the other was inactive and had a higher percentage of fat – let's call him Barney – and fed them both a diet of 3,000 calories per day, Fred is likely to metabolize or burn those calories just by carrying out the everyday processes of growth and repair. Barney, on the other hand, will not need as many calories, as he has less muscle tissue to maintain, so he adds to his excess stores of fat daily. The rate at which he adds to his fat stores will continue to increase all the time he doesn't exercise, and the fat percentage of his body weight will go up and up.

Genetic factors also determine to some extent the amount of fat you carry on your body. However if a couple who are overweight have a child, it is likely to become overweight because it will be eating the same diet as its parents, not because of its genetic inheritance. Many people use their genes as a reason for being overweight, but in reality if you do inherit excessive fat cells (which is rare) you will only become overweight if you decide to fill them up with fat!

If I am asked to put into one sentence the best way to lose weight, I always say: 'Eat more vegetables and fruit, eat less meat and fewer dairy products and exercise regularly.' There are very few people for whom this formula doesn't work. In fact I can honestly say that I don't know anyone who has stuck to this method and not lost weight and improved their body shape.

FAT IS FAT – ISN'T IT?

Fat is a very topical issue, but the information and advice currently in the media are often conflicting! Many perceive all fat as 'bad' and are damaging their health in trying to follow a low-fat or, worse still, no-fat diet. There are many 'good' fats that will make your body strong and healthy, and will help you to withstand disease and illness. In addition to this, they will actually help your body to metabolize or burn other fats, which is crucial if you want to lose weight and change your shape. All fats are not equal.

As we have seen, not all fat stored on the body is surplus to requirement. Fat acts as a protective blanket which shields us from cold and other traumas. Fatty deposits also hold our organs in place. I remember clearly when I was studying and we dissected a lamb's kidney. When the tutor brought it out of the bag it was basically just a blob of white fat, no sight of a kidney at all, but when she cut through it, the kidney literally slid out of the middle of this protective sheath, like a marble out of a bag. Of course the kidney is such an important organ, it has to be protected from damage and the fatty sheath does exactly that. It is not only the kidneys that are protected in this way, but all of our vital organs. In addition, a large proportion of our brain is made up of fat and fat also plays a vital role in our nervous system.

Fats which are essential for normal metabolism are called essential fatty acids (EFAs). In fact they are thought to increase the metabolic rate, as opposed to saturated fats (fats that are solid at room and body temperature, e.g. animal fats), which are thought to slow the metabolic rate down.

GETTING THE BALANCE RIGHT

Too much body fat leads to obesity, which increases your risk of disease, but too little body fat can also be a problem, particularly for females, for if the body fat levels drop too low, as mentioned earlier, menstruation ceases, which adversely affects hormone levels in the body and can lead to osteoporosis, infertility and other problems. Clearly we need to find a middle ground.

If your diet is made up primarily of vegetables and fruit, with limited dairy products, but including fish and some seeds, you will automatically be achieving the correct balance of nutrients required for vitality and for maintaining the desired level of body fat.

It may sound corny, but we really are what we eat. Every single living cell in your body is made from the foods that you eat. If you fill yourself up with foods that have been over-processed and refined, instead of providing your body with all the nutrients it needs for anabolism, that is, building up body tissues, you are putting in foods that can actually disrupt this vital metabolic process. It is hardly surprising that if we don't supply our body with good quality materials, the cells it builds are second or even third rate. We feel lethargic, constantly tired, develop skin problems such as acne or dry patches, or persistent coughs that won't go away and numerous other unpleasant symptoms, all because we are not giving our bodies the right material to do the job.

Let's look now at all the different types of fat and then discuss each one in more detail.

Table 4: ***Fat Chart***

Saturated Fats	*Monounsaturated Fats*	*Polyunsaturated Fats*
beef	olive oil	soyabean
pork	canola oil	safflower
lamb	almond oil	sunflower
poultry		corn
coconut oil		sesame
milk		
dairy produce		
palm oil		

Linoleic Acid (Omega 6)	*Linolenic Acid (Omega 3)*
soyabean	flaxseed (linseed)
safflower	soyabean
sunflower	rapeseed (canola)
corn	pumpkin
wheatgerm	walnut
sesame	fish
evening primrose oil	

WHAT IS A SATURATED FAT?

When you hear all the different names there are for different types of fats and fatty acids, you could be forgiven for getting quite confused. I certainly have done – many times! But in reality, it can be simplified quite easily.

You will find saturated fatty acids (SFAs) in all foods, fats and oils to a greater or lesser extent, but they are most abundant in hard fats, that is, fats that are solid at room and body temperature. These fats are simplest in structure and are the ones that cause us the most health problems. Just remember next time you eat a fat that is solid at room temperature that once it is in your body it will become solid again. Don't think just because it is liquid whilst you are cooking with it, it will stay liquid. It is because of this that it literally clogs up arteries!

In the blood SFAs stick together to form large fat globules. If you ate a cheeseburger and a milkshake and then immediately took a blood sample, within about an hour you would see that your blood had almost completely congealed and solidified. Imagine how hard your body has to work to constantly break down and digest all these solid fats.

Sometimes, of course, the large fat globules in the blood can ultimately lead to a clot large enough to block an artery. Obviously this is a major health risk and we should therefore restrict our intake of these hard fats by reducing the amount of meat, in particular beef, mutton/lamb and pork, and all dairy produce in our diet. It is also worth remembering that our body converts excess sugar into SFAs, as explained earlier.

Eating saturated fat can have dire consequences if you are trying to lose weight, first because it will solidify in your body and secondly because it will slow down your metabolism, preventing you from burning calories. A diet which is high in saturated fats is more likely to make you feel lazy and lethargic, whereas a diet that contains lots of vegetables and fruit and very little meat will ensure that you are getting the optimum amount of nutrients and give you more energy. You will feel like a new person – and very soon you will have a new shape to go with it.

UNSATURATED FATTY ACIDS (UFAS)

If saturated fats are solid at room temperature, unsaturated fatty acids (UFAs) are liquid. They have a different structure from SFAs which changes the shape of the fatty acid completely. If you looked at a UFA under a microscope it would look like a bendy caterpillar, whereas a SFA would look more like a stick. This means they behave differently in the body. One important factor is that UFAs don't stick together like SFAs. In fact they positively push each other apart. This is very important as it means they are not likely to form blood clots. It also means that they are able to undertake many other important functions in the body without always getting stuck together.

The fats that we should be increasing in our diet are the *unsaturated essential fatty acids*, or EFAs. They are called 'essential' because the body cannot make them itself. Deficiency of these vital oils can lead to many problems, including:

high blood pressure
PMS or breast pain
eczema or dry skin
dry eyes
inflammatory problems, e.g. arthritis
water retention
tingling in the arms and legs
being prone to infection
decline in memory or learning ability
lack of co-ordination or impaired vision

Diseases which affect the nervous system, such as multiple sclerosis, have been linked to deficiencies in certain EFAs. Many sufferers of such diseases have experienced long periods of remission and drastically slowed down the progress of the disease using nutritional therapy.

The unsaturated fatty acid group can be further broken down into:

*Monounsaturated fatty acids (MUFAs)*MUFAs are rather a mixed bag. Some are found in milk, coconut and palm oil, (even though coconut and palm oil are also highly saturated) which interfere with the conversion of other EFAs. There are, however, longer chain MUFAs which are beneficial to health. These are found in olive, almond, canola and other oils. They help to keep our arteries supple.

Linoleic acid (omega 6) and alpha linolenic acid (omega 3)
These unsaturated fatty acids are extremely beneficial in terms of health and we *must* obtain them from our diet in order to stay healthy. They make up vital components in all cells, in particular brain and nerve cells. Our body also uses these substances to make prostaglandins. These are tiny hormone-like structures which regulate many functions in the cells. Unfortunately they are very short lived and as we cannot store vast reserves of them we have to be able to constantly manufacture them from EFAs.

PROSTAGLANDINS – VITAL FOR HEALTH

There are many different types of prostaglandins with many different functions, including preventing blood platelets sticking together, removing excess sodium and fluid from our kidneys, improving circulation and lowering blood pressure. They have also been linked to reducing and regulating cholesterol production and helping conditions such as arthritis. They also help insulin work more effectively, thereby helping diabetics, improve nerve function, regulate calcium metabolism and improve the efficiency of our immune system. As you can see, they have plenty of work to do in the body, therefore we must give our body all the nutrients it needs to be able to manufacture new prostaglandins all the time.

When we are in good health and eating a balanced diet, our body is able to make all the prostaglandins it needs. However, there are some things that we eat that actually prevent the body from converting EFAs into prostaglandins. This is where nutritional supplements such as evening primrose oil can be useful. They have already undergone the first steps of conversion, therefore we can literally bypass some of the processing stages and take something much closer to the end product. However, you should always look to your food as the primary source of nutrients. After all we can't live off capsules and supplements alone.

THE AMOUNT AND QUALITY OF FAT

Our level of fat intake is directly related to our weight. But it is not just the amount of fat we eat that determines our health, but where we get the fats from. As already mentioned, it is possible to have a diet high in saturated fats and still be deficient in EFAs. If we take in adequate supplies of linoleic and alpha linolenic acid, however, and have a diet rich in vitamins and minerals, we can make all the EFAs we need.

In the UK the average diet is thought to contain over 45 per cent of fat calories. This is way over most nutritional guidelines, which vary between 10 and 30 per cent. Bear in mind that most of these fat calories come from saturated and other poor quality fats, which not only cause you to gain weight, but are more likely to put you at risk of suffering from heart disease or cancer. My main concern is the *quality* of the fat you are eating. Yet even the essential omega 3 and omega 6 fats need make up only 3–5 per cent of our total calorific intake.

Here are a few tips to help you reduce the saturated content of your diet without reducing your intake of EFAs:

Eat more vegetables (some raw if possible).
Eat more fruit, especially in place of cakes and pastries, etc.
Eat less meat, in particular red meat and offal.
When you do use meat, trim off all excess fat or skin before cooking.
Do not use saturated fats for cooking. Replace with oils such as extra virgin olive oil and use only a tiny amount.
Reduce the amount of dairy produce you eat.
Use skimmed milk instead of full cream or semi skimmed.
Bake or grill foods instead of frying.
Eat more wholegrains, such as cereals, e.g. rye, oats, brown rice and corn.
Choose low-fat sources of protein, such as fish, turkey, chicken or dried peas or beans (legumes).

OIL SUPPLEMENTS

Several different oil supplements have come onto the market recently. Here are the main ones.

Evening Primrose Oil

Evening primrose oil is probably the best documented of these oils. It comes from the seeds of the evening primrose plant and contains high levels of linolenic oil. The evening primrose plant has been used for healing purposes for many years in North America, but only recently has its therapeutic value been appreciated internationally. This is due in part to the progress scientists have made in extracting the valuable oil from the seeds.

Studies with EPO have suggested that it may help with many conditions. It has a role in lowering blood pressure and cholesterol levels, thereby reducing the risk of suffering a stroke or heart attack, helping weight loss by increasing the metabolic rate, relieving premenstrual tension and breast pain, easing certain kinds of eczema and improving the condition of the hair and nails.

I have met many people who have said that taking EPO has literally changed their life, they feel so much better. This may be true, but you must also look at your diet as well and not just into a pill bottle. The meals in this book are a good start – they are all well balanced and contain not just all the essential fats that your body needs, but also the other vital nutrients as well.

Fish Oils

Fish oils come, obviously, from fish, but the fish that

are richest in EFAs are cold water fish, such as salmon, sardines, mackerel, trout, herring and eel. When you have eaten these fish, it takes your body two to three weeks to metabolize the EFAs into usable form, therefore you should eat fish once a fortnight at the very least. I remember from my school dinners that Friday was fish day! Now I understand why.

When preparing fish, you should boil or poach it rather than fry it. This is because frying can destroy some of the EFAs you are trying to consume. In Japan fish is eaten raw. Although this may sound unusual, at least it preserves the valuable oils.

Fish oils are thought to have the following health benefits: they prevent blood platelets from becoming too sticky, thereby reducing the risk of a clot causing a stroke or heart attack, help maintain the structure of the arteries, reduce blood triglyceride levels, reduce blood pressure and help to make prostaglandins. In some cases fish oils have been linked to the slowing down or prevention of the growth of cancer tumours. There are also other EFAs that may be equally or even more beneficial. If you are interested in learning more about the fats we eat, then I recommend *Fats That Heal, Fats That Kill* by Udo Erasmus (Alive Books, 1993).

HOW FAT IS BROKEN DOWN IN THE BODY

How many times have you heard the saying 'If you eat that, it will go straight to your hips' or 'A moment on the lips, a lifetime on the hips'? Well, it's not exactly true, the fat you eat doesn't go *straight* to your hips, although it may end up there. Like any other food it has to be broken down and digested, and where it ends up depends on how much you have eaten and your activity level.

DIGESTION

The process of fat digestion begins in the mouth. As you chew, you start to break down and separate the fats before you swallow.

The food then goes into the stomach. Not much happens to it here, apart from the fact that it is broken down into smaller pieces. The stomach contains hydrochloric acid, which breaks down protein, but any fat eaten with protein must wait until it reaches the intestines before it can begin to be fully digested and absorbed. The enzymes involved in breaking down fat come from the pancreas.

The Gall Bladder

The gall bladder plays an important role in fat digestion, as it supplies the bile which emulsifies the fats, breaking them down into tiny droplets. The bile is like washing up liquid, breaking down the greasy food molecules into smaller and smaller droplets. Without washing up liquid, water alone cannot break down the fats on greasy plates and dishes. Fat digestion uses bile in exactly the same way.

The gall bladder is an extension of the liver. Bile is manufactured in the liver and then concentrated and stored in the gall bladder. People who have had their gall bladder removed (often due to a diet which has been too high in fats) can still digest fat, but the bile they produce is more diluted and therefore not so effective.

Absorbing Fat

Fats are ultimately digested and absorbed in the intestines. But once they have been broken down completely and absorbed through the gut wall, they are put back together again. It seems a little strange that we break foods down only to put them back together again! But actually this process is vital, as it ensures that we don't absorb any tissues or other unwanted substance by literally taking it apart to make sure we only absorb what we want. It's just like taking a puzzle to pieces and making it again, but in the shapes we can use best. In other words, we adapt the shape of the molecules we eat to form shapes that our body can use more readily. Your body absorbs all foods in this way.

Some unnatural processed foods, however, such as hydrogenated fats, cannot be broken down and rebuilt, so they stay in their chemically altered unnatural shape, even after they have been absorbed. When the body tries to use these fats, it causes problems, because they don't 'fit' into any of our body's mechanisms. It's like trying to fit a square peg into a round hole. This can lead to the destruction of many vital cell structures. More on hydrogenated fats later.

Once the absorption of fats is complete, they are carried off in specialized sacs in the lymph vessels to a blood vessel close to the heart that merges with the normal circulation system, rather like a slip road onto the motorway. In this way the fat is literally dropped off and can be carried in the blood either to be metabolized to provide energy or for some other function. If we have taken in more than we need it goes to the fat cells to be stored.

FAT REPLACEMENTS

Fats add a great deal of flavour to our food – after all, if they tasted awful we wouldn't have a problem in not eating them, would we?! So, with 'low-fat phobia', chemists have been under pressure to come up with fat substitutes. They have to be of similar texture and flavour to fat, but contain fewer calories. Several companies have now produced products that fit this description, many of which we can find in processed foods.

The problems associated with these replacement fat substances are not yet known, as the process is still very new. However, people are now seduced into thinking that they are making healthy choices by eating these products, which are typically high in refined sugars and low in fibre. Unfortunately, many unscrupulous advertising companies will twist and turn any facts into half-truths and miss out key information in order to entice us into buying their products. I despair when I see foods advertised as 'healthy alternatives' that are really made up from over-processed, nutrient-empty substances that do not only not provide vitamins and minerals, but often contain substances that actually block the absorption of nutrients we have eaten.

At least one product, olestra, has now been cleared for use in some snack foods that resembles fat in every sense, except that it is not digested by the body and therefore passes through relatively unchanged, rather like fibre. The problem is that in going through the body it absorbs other valuable nutrients, which are then expelled by the body instead of being used.It can also lead to very weak bowels and incontinence. I recently heard Udo Erasmus, a leading expert on fats, saying that if these products become widely available, we should all invest in the nappy industry!

Remember, low-fat varieties of processed foods don't stop you eating junk food – you are just eating a different type of junk food. The real answer is to eat more natural foods, i.e. *naturally* low-fat foods which contain no refined products, just bundles of nutrients. Why look to packet foods when nature provides the best alternative?

CHOLESTEROL – GOOD OR BAD?

It would be wrong to discuss fat without mentioning cholesterol. Like fat, it has a bad reputation but is essential for life. It is also clear, however, that there is a definite link between high levels of cholesterol and cardiovascular disease (CVD).

The subject of cholesterol is possibly even more controversial than that of fat itself. First we must ask the question: 'What is cholesterol and just how much do we really need?'

Cholesterol is a hard waxy substance. We do need it and can get it directly from the diet, *but* our body is able to manufacture it itself. In other words, even if you never eat any cholesterol-containing foods again, your body will be able to make all you need, providing your diet contains some carbohydrate, some fats and some protein. The more calories you consume, the more cholesterol your body will make. Therefore, people who overeat generally manufacture more cholesterol than they need. This is when it becomes harmful.

Cholesterol in the diet comes from animal sources. All plant foods, i.e. carbohydrates, are cholesterol free. Foods containing cholesterol include:

eggs
meat
dairy products
fish
shellfish

GOOD *AND* BAD CHOLESTEROL

Cholesterol is carried around the body in two different forms, HDL (high density lipoproteins) and LDL (low density lipoproteins). These molecules work in opposite ways: LDL transports cholesterol around the body and deposits excess in the arteries, and HDL comes along, mops up the excess and takes it to the liver, where it can be broken down and disposed of. It is not just the amount of cholesterol that you have that is significant in terms of health, but the ratio of HDL to LDL.

WHY WE NEED IT

Our body uses cholesterol for many different reasons. Its primary function is to help maintain the normal structure of our cells. If a cell membrane is too stiff and rigid, it will stop nutrients and waste products from getting in and out of the cell, and so the body will remove some cholesterol from this particular structure. If, on the other hand, the membrane is too sloppy, cholesterol can be added.

Our body also makes the steroid hormones from cholesterol. Thank goodness for that, as these are the hormones that make men different from women and vice versa!

Other valuable hormones are also made from cholesterol, including those that help to maintain water balance in the body, prepare glucose in response to stress and suppress inflammation. Vitamin D, which is essential for calcium metabolism, is manufactured from it. Bile acids, mentioned earlier in the digestive process, are also composed in part of cholesterol.

Excess cholesterol is removed in the process of excretion along with the other unwanted solid substances. It is in this way that cholesterol helps to break down other fats in the body.

Cholesterol is also secreted by glands in our skin. It stops the skin from drying out and cracking. It also helps protect against sunlight, wind and water, and unwanted invading organisms.

ALCOHOL AND CHOLESTEROL

If you consume large amounts of alcohol, then the body makes more cholesterol. The reason for this may be that alcohol makes our cell membranes more runny. As mentioned before, when this happens more cholesterol has to be added to the membrane to restore its structure. Once the alcohol wears off, the membrane starts to harden, leaving a surplus of cholesterol which is then dumped into the blood. It travels to the liver where it becomes part of bile acids, which, providing there are sufficient nutrients and fibre in the diet, will be eliminated along with the body's normal waste. With insufficient fibre or irregular bowel movements, however, the cholesterol is not eliminated and can be reabsorbed.

MAKING EXCESS CHOLESTEROL

In most people, the body can recognize when the dietary intake of cholesterol is too high and cut back on its own cholesterol production to compensate. In some people, however, this natural feedback system does not work, which can lead to incredibly high levels of cholesterol in the blood. The daily turnover of cholesterol in the average person is approximately 1 gram (0.03 oz). This figure is lower in strict vegetarians.

Once you have made excess cholesterol, it can't be turned into anything else. Therefore you have to get rid of it. As already mentioned, excess cholesterol is removed in the process of excretion, along with the other unwanted solid substances. This removal process is more efficient if you are taking in adequate quantities of fibre. If not, your body can reabsorb as much as 90 per cent of the cholesterol.

FAT AND YOUR HEART

The way in which cholesterol can be most harmful to our health is through our blood vessels. Healthy blood vessels are essential to transport blood around the body. The 'head office' for this system is the heart. All blood flows either to or from the heart.

When you breathe in, the oxygen you breathe goes into the lungs, where it dissolves into the blood via tiny structures called alveoli. The blood flows from the alveoli to the heart and then begins a one-way journey around the body, with oxygen diffusing out of the blood vessels constantly.

The blood vessels that leave the heart carrying all this energy-giving, oxygenated blood are called arteries. They get smaller and smaller as they spread out, just like a road network, leading ultimately to the cells. Once all the oxygen has been diffused, the blood returns to the heart via the system of veins. Then it is sent back to the lungs to collect more oxygen and the whole one-way cycle is complete, and thankfully continuous! In this way the whole body is supplied with all the nutrients it needs, providing there are no blockages in the system.

The heart itself has its own circulation system, as it requires large amounts of oxygen to function. After all, it is the muscle that can never rest. It is in this system that blockages most often occur. The arteries that supply the heart are called coronary arteries. Like other arteries, these get smaller and smaller as they reach their destination. If these arteries become blocked, an area of the heart muscle is starved of oxygen, which means it cannot function. That area of muscle tissue then dies and cannot be repaired. Providing this affects only a small area of the heart, the patient can make a good recovery and should be encouraged to take up some form of controlled exercise regime in order to strengthen the remaining healthy muscle tissue, so that it can cope more efficiently and reduce the risks of further clots forming. However, if the blockage is in one of the main coronary arteries, a large area of the heart muscle is starved of oxygen and this can be fatal. The same thing applies in principle to the brain, where a blockage may cause a stroke.

You can see how important it is to monitor the amount of saturated fatty acids and cholesterol in the diet in order to minimize the likelihood of clots forming. Do not forget that exercise plays a key role in the prevention of heart disease as well *(see Chapter 7)*.

HYDROGENATED OILS

As I mentioned earlier, another kind of fat that is potentially harmful to health is hydrogenated fat. You may have heard this term – it refers to the process of turning liquid oils into hard or solid fats, or even plastics. This is done by heating the oils to a very high temperature and chemically changing the structure of the fat molecules, which involves breaking down the double bonds in the fatty acids and replacing them with hydrogen bonds, hence the name 'hydrogenation'. Metals are also used in this process, such as nickel and aluminium, and remnants of these can be found in the hydrogenated oils or fats which we eat.

AN UNNATURAL SUBSTANCE

We are part of nature and it never ceases to amaze me how the circle of life involves almost every species. The sun enables the plants to grow and we eat the plants or the animals that have eaten the plants. Either way, our energy comes ultimately from the sun and the plants. This is the natural process of feeding the human body. Everything has been perfectly designed to fit into the complicated jigsaw of life.

We are able to break down natural substances; however, we are not designed to be able to break down man-made foreign substances, such as hydrogenated fats. Remember, absorbing hydrogenated fat is like trying to fit a square peg into a round hole. It won't fit. If you try to force it, you will cause damage to the structure, and that is exactly what happens in your body. Consumption of hydrogenated fat has been linked to cancer and other diseases.

Hydrogenated oils are used in products such as chocolate. They enable it to stay relatively solid in its packaging and yet still to melt in the mouth (liquid fat – sounds awful, doesn't it?) Products that include partially hydrogenated fats include margarines and shortenings.

Industry's reason for using the hydrogenation process is that it provides cheap spreadable products for consumer consumption. But you should consider the effect these unnatural products have on your health. I certainly don't want to put them into my body.

TRANS FATTY ACIDS

Margarines and shortenings also contain large quantities of trans fatty acids. These fatty acids are produced by high temperatures and the process of hydrogenation and also interfere with health by blocking normal biological processes.

Margarines contribute the bulk of all trans fatty acids consumed in the Western diet. It is interesting to note, however, that the Dutch Government has now banned the sale of hydrogenated margarines and other foods containing trans fatty acids, and the research showing their adverse effects is quite clear. Perhaps we will eventually have the same warning on products containing hydrogenated oils as we do on cigarettes!

Some companies are now using more 'normal' (cis) fatty acids in their margarines, and these are good, so always check the labels. What makes a trans fatty acid different from a cis fatty acid is that it is twisted in its make up. A cis fatty acid is U-shaped, whereas a trans fatty acid is bent and twisted in the centre. It looks a little like a rag that has been wrung out in the middle.

Although this change isn't that extreme in terms of structure, it does drastically change how the molecule behaves in our body. Think of it as a piece of a jigsaw that has been cut to the wrong shape. In the same way as a faulty jigsaw piece, the trans fatty acids in our body do not fit the hole. Unfortunately, they take up enough of the hole to stop the normal (cis) fatty acid from getting in. So they can adversely affect the cell membrane, letting into the cell some molecules that should be kept out and letting out some that should be kept in. If the cell membrane is weakened in this way, cancers are more likely to form. Trans fatty acids have been associated with many forms of cancer.

Another characteristic of trans fatty acids is that they are very sticky, which makes them more likely to cause a blood clot.

Cutting Down

You can decrease the amount of trans fatty acids you consume by reading food labels more carefully. If you see that the product contains hydrogenated oils, then the chances are it will also be high in trans fatty acids.

Products such as crisps and most confectionery will contain hydrogenated oils, so there is good reason not to eat them even if you are not on a weight loss programme.

WHERE DOES THE FAT IN *YOUR* DIET COME FROM?

Every food that is living contains fat. That is because fats make up the cell membranes of all living things. But what type of fat are you eating and how much?

If you eat lots of processed foods, such as pies, pasties, sausages, burgers, chocolate and other confectionery such as ice cream, etc., then your diet is certainly very high in fat. Not only that, it is very high in saturated fats and low in the vital unsaturated fats which contain the EFAs. I rarely find that someone who eats a pasty or a meat and potato pie for tea serves it with fresh broccoli and carrots, so the amount of carbohydrate is also often lower than the amount of fat consumed. In the Western world, this kind of diet is very common. So are the degenerative diseases associated with a lack of EFAs and other essential nutrients, such as heart disease, cancer and many others. A possible link? In my opinion it is not only possible but obvious. Besides, if you examine diets from other areas of the world that don't contain so many processed foods, you will find the incidence of degenerative disease drastically lower and in some cases non-existent.

So how can you increase your consumption of the beneficial EFAs while decreasing the amount of harmful fat in your diet? I'm sure you get the idea by now: more vegetables, fruit, wholegrains, cereals and seeds!

In vegetables, the greenest part of the plant contains the most EFAs. These EFAs unfortunately degenerate when the plant has been picked, therefore fresh vegetables contain more. Cooking also destroys many of the nutrients. Vitamin C levels are reduced by as much as 50 per cent during cooking. Oils from plants contain almost no cholesterol.

Fruit also contains some fats, about the same amount as the non-green part of plants.

Legumes also contain some EFAs, although the amount varies. Examples of legumes that contain EFAs include lentils, peas, mung and lima beans, chick peas and soyabeans. Surprisingly, peanuts are also classified as legumes (because they are more pea than nut!) but, contrary to popular opinion, nutritionally they are very poor.

USEFUL TIPS

Always keep your vegetable water to use as stock in stews or soups, or to make gravy. I regularly throw all my vegetables into a large pan, simmer them for about 30 minutes and then blend them into soup. This makes a wonderfully delicious meal that also freezes well and is economical. I usually have two or three bowls of soup in the freezer and when I come home from work in the evening it only takes a few minutes to heat one through. The only fats contained in the soup are the natural ones found in the vegetables. A few seeds or ground almonds can also be added before blending for a slightly different taste.

Sesame oil can be useful in cooking – a tiny

amount in stir fries will give a really nice taste. Use a pastry brush to spread a teaspoonful of the oil around your wok or large frying pan. Make sure you stir the food continually, so that it all comes in contact with the oil. If you are cooking for two people or just for one, use half a teaspoonful.

Most legumes retain their nutrients whilst they are cooking, but these nutrients deteriorate after cooking, so try to eat the food as quickly as possible.

Oils in nuts and seeds are protected from the damaging effects of heat, light and oxygen by their hard cases or shells. Once these shells have been broken, the fats deteriorate and go rancid, so only eat fresh nuts and seeds.

DAIRY PRODUCE

Many dairy products contain some trans fatty acids. As they are of animal origin they also contain high levels of saturated fat. The quality of the fat that we get from dairy products is dependent on the feed given to the animal. For example, if the cow is fed antibiotics when it is ill, as many are, they may ultimately end up in our digestive system when we drink the milk or eat the meat. This can lead to digestive problems, which may in turn cause food intolerances or allergies. If the digestive process is impaired, foods are not properly absorbed. This leads to nutrient deficiencies which will in turn lead to other problems. If your digestive system is not functioning properly, it is possible to eat all the nutrients you require, but not absorb them. People who eat a diet high in wholefoods, natural grains, lots of vegetables and fruit, limited amounts of dairy products and refined foods rarely suffer from these kinds of problems.

Eggs can also vary in their nutrient content according to the quality of the chicken feed. A poor quality feed will lead to a poor quality egg. Organically fed, free range chickens generally produce much healthier and certainly tastier eggs. The white contains no fat at all. The yolk is where the fat is contained. It also contains about 250 mg (0.0075 oz) of cholesterol. Eggs are fine if eaten in moderation. I certainly don't hold with the phrase 'Go to work on an egg', but I do enjoy a really tasty free range egg from time to time.

BUTTER OR MARGARINE?

There is huge debate as to whether butter or margarine is better for you. Let's look at the merits and disadvantages of each in turn.

Butter

One of the problems with butter is that, unlike most natural foods, it does not contain the nutrients required for its own digestion, therefore these have to be taken from other foods eaten. Also, as with milk, antibiotics, hormones or any other chemicals given to the animal can ultimately end up on our toast!

Butter generally contains about 6 per cent trans fatty acids, which is a relatively low level. A pound (0.4 kg) of butter contains about 1 gram (0.03 oz) of cholesterol. One of the benefits butter has over other fats is that it can withstand moderate temperatures, although if the temperature is too high the protein in the butter turns black. It can also stand light and oxygen. This makes it fairly safe for cooking and baking.

I would say that although butter isn't exactly good for you, it isn't that bad, in moderation. Obviously I would advise against lashings on bread or jacket potatoes. Butter has quite a strong taste and a little goes a long way. Try buttering only one slice of bread in a sandwich if you want to cut down but can't face the dryness of bread without a spread.

Margarine

Margarines are constantly changing. Most contain hydrogenated fats (check the label and you will see). These compete with the EFAs that may have been present and can cause problems.

As with butter, margarine does not contain the nutrients it requires for its own breakdown and digestion, and may contain antibiotics, depending on the source. Unlike butter, it is *not* suitable for frying or cooking at high temperatures because of its water content. Margarine contains up to 20 per cent water, which over a period of time affects the structure of the double bonds, slowly destroying them. It is also affected by heat, light and oxygen, which all adversely change its structure.

You may see margarines advertised as containing polyunsaturated fats, which are usually good. However these have usually been chemically manufactured and are therefore not good.

It is possible to make margarine without trans fatty acids, but in the UK these unhydrogenated spreads are not generally available.

If you want to put a completely unnatural, over-processed substance on your bread, then margarine is for you! If not, I advise you to stick to small amounts of butter or nothing at all.

KNOW WHAT YOU EAT

Over the past two or three years my own diet has changed considerably. Now when I eat something, I want to know what it is going to do to my body. Will it enhance my state of health or will it be detrimental? Everything you eat will have either a positive or negative effect on your health and the general day-to-day running of your body.

Whilst I have developed a passion for knowing what goes on inside my body, I appreciate that not everyone wants to go to such great lengths, so you can choose to what extent you want to make changes. I would encourage you, however, to think about the health consequences, both good and bad, of what you eat, and not just whether or not it will cause you to gain weight.

Don't Worry

I have designed the recipes in this book not just to help you to lose weight, but also to incorporate all the information I have given here, so don't worry if you don't understand or can't remember some of it. If you follow the recipes and the general guidelines, you will automatically be getting it right. Not only will you lose weight, but you will also be providing your body with an abundance of nutrients that it will use to build and repair your ever-changing cells. You will have more energy, your skin and hair will improve, and on the inside, all of your body's systems that work so wonderfully and intricately together will be able to function in perfect harmony. You will literally start to glow with renewed health and vitality!

Chapter 6

Detoxification – Spring Cleaning

The body produces toxins every day as it goes about its many normal biochemical functions. It has several ways of handling these toxins and expelling them. Providing our systems are functioning efficiently, they do not cause us a problem. If we reach a state where our body cannot get rid of the toxins as fast as we are making them, however, we are in a state of toxicity. The problem is that we not only have to cope with the toxins that our body produces, but also with extra toxins that we eat, drink and inhale on a daily basis. The air today contains many new and far stronger chemicals than ever before. Also, many drugs and food additives can create toxic elements in the body. If these excess toxins are not eliminated, they cause irritation and inflammation of our cells and body tissues. They also block normal metabolic functions in individual cells, which affects our organs and ultimately our whole body.

If you are serious about wanting to lose weight, then the first step is to look at what you eat, not only the foods that have caused you to gain weight, but also the foods that may be stopping your digestion from functioning efficiently and thereby preventing you from losing weight. In other words, you need to give your digestive system a spring clean.

WHAT IS A SPRING CLEAN?

It is a three-day programme that will ensure that you get the best possible start. It contains only foods from the most natural sources. Many are uncooked and therefore rich in nutrients that will help to give you a boost and get rid of some of the toxins that may have been building up in your body over many years. It will not only help you to lose weight, but also to restore yourself to good health. You may want to repeat this once a month, to keep your digestive system clean and healthy.

This is only a very short programme. Many people follow this kind of regime for much longer.

Some of you may find you lose several pounds over the first few days, others may lose much smaller amounts. The purpose of the spring clean is not just to lose weight, but to cleanse the digestive system and make sure that everything is functioning properly. Therefore, don't weigh yourself until you have followed the programme for a full week at least. Preferably two. Some people take longer to get their body into a state where it can burn off excess calories more easily than others. It's much better to judge your success by how loose your clothes begin to feel and how much more energy you have than by the scales alone.

During the spring clean, you must drink as much water as possible to help your body flush out the toxins that you will be releasing.

HUNGER PANGS

You may feel hungry; you may even really crave food. Rest assured you will be getting all the nutrients you require and the craving is not coming from a genuine need for food but from a false hunger, caused by years of eating refined foods *(see pages 6 and 39)*.

In spite of this, it is very important that you stick to the spring clean for the full three days. You must not give in to desires for sweet things, however strong. Think of these desires as ghosts of foods past, coming back to haunt you and tempt you into breaking this vital first step on your weight loss programme. You *are* going to be successful, you *are* going to lose weight, you *are* going to lose inches, you *are* going to have much more energy, but you are *not* going to achieve these things if you fall at the first hurdle. Jump that hurdle.

Anyone can follow this spring clean and benefit, irrespective of whether or not they want to lose weight. Why not get your partner or a friend to do it with you? Then you can both feel great.

GETTING RID OF THE RUBBISH

If your diet has been extremely high in refined and processed foods, then as your tissues give up their store of toxins and release them into the blood to be disposed of, you may feel a little groggy. You may have headaches and feel generally low. These are classic withdrawal symptoms. Persevere – they will be gone in three days.

Don't worry if you feel irritable or even sleepless

the first few days. This is because your body is working hard to expel the toxins. The body does a lot of its detoxifying overnight, which is why people often wake up feeling nauseous and feel better as the day progresses.

Unlike the drug addict, whose symptoms of withdrawal can be very long lasting, the body gets rid of toxins very quickly, given the chance. As long as you drink lots of water, your organs can literally flush all the rubbish out.

FEELING GREAT

By the time you finish the spring clean, you will be starting to feel wonderful. As you progress onto the other recipes, your health and energy levels will be going up and up every day. The headaches will be gone.

After a few weeks you may notice an improvement in your skin and complexion, your hair and your nails. You will be losing body fat at a steady rate and you will look and feel great. If you follow the recipes and the exercises in this programme, it *will* work. No false promises! The truth is, anyone who eats healthily becomes healthy.

TEA AND COFFEE

If you drink tea and coffee, I suggest you reduce these as much as possible over a period of several days *before* the spring clean. They are stimulants and if you drink more than two or three cups per day, particularly of coffee, you need to wean yourself off prior to the spring clean. Your body will not benefit from it if you continue to have them. The problem with giving up tea and coffee in one go is that it can leave you with a severe headache, which will last until your body has eliminated all the toxins they have caused. This normally takes three to five days.

Once you have completed the spring clean, you may wish to reintroduce these drinks (although I wouldn't recommend it!) If you feel you really can't do without your caffeine fix, then at least try to restrict the amount you drink. You should also note that if you drink tea or coffee within an hour of eating, the amount of nutrients (in particular vitamin C) that your body can absorb is reduced by as much as 60 per cent. Instead, have a glass of water before your meal and sip it throughout if you feel thirsty. Save tea and coffee until later.

I was speaking to a member of my club recently who was telling me he drinks up to 30 cups of coffee per day. This is because it is literally on tap where he works. At the weekend, when he is at home, he has one cup in the morning and that is all. He always suffers a headache by Sunday, which goes as soon as he has his coffee fix on a Monday, but he had never linked the two. He is giving his liver so much extra work, constantly building up stores of toxins, as the body can't possibly excrete this amount of waste. These toxins are stored in body tissues and when he doesn't have coffee they have a chance to release them. Although the coffee relieves the headache in the short term, in the long term he is adding to the already serious problem. I have advised him to reduce his coffee by two or three cups per day rather than give it up all together. For him, it will be a slow process. He will have to go at his own pace. But his ultimate goal, now he knows the perils, is to give it up completely.

GETTING STARTED

You must decide when is the best time to begin your programme. Although most people like to start a 'diet' on a Monday, I recommend a Friday if you work a normal week. This will mean you can complete the spring clean without being exposed to coffee machines, vending machines and other temptations that you may have at work. If you do start on a Monday, make sure you plan your food according to the menu.

Is It Important to Start with the Spring Clean?
If possible, yes. However if you feel you cannot manage it, then don't worry, just go on to the other recipes. There are a few people who the spring clean may not suit or it may be impractical for you to do it at this time. If this is the case, do try and do it at some time in the future, as your body will really benefit.

THE TLC THREE-DAY SPRING CLEAN DIET

This is the first step of your weight loss programme. As already explained, it really will give you the best possible start by allowing your body – and in particular your digestive system – to clean out some of the toxins it has been storing.

The spring clean lasts for three days. You may choose from the breakfast, lunch and dinner recipes – it doesn't matter which order you have the meals in.

You may prefer to have the same thing for breakfast each day, similarly with lunch and dinner. You may find that if you have made a large pot of soup, for example, there is enough for three days. The aim of the recipes is to provide you with three days of natural foods, with no dairy produce, meat or additives of any kind. Bread or wheat products are also excluded. Everything you eat during these three days must be fresh and completely unprocessed or unrefined.

I have not put the amount or weight of any foods, as providing you stick those suggested, you can eat as much as you like.

BREAKFAST

= Fruit and diluted fruit juice.

Choose fruit that you like to eat. Make sure you wash and peel any with skin on. You may wish to make a fresh fruit salad *(see page 167)* or prefer to eat pieces of fruit individually. Whichever you prefer is fine.

N.B. If you suffer from arthritis, you should avoid citrus fruit.

LUNCH

= Soup.

Choose from the soups on pages 172–4. I have indicated which ones are suitable for the spring clean. Have two bowls if one does not satisfy you.

DINNER

= Salad and jacket potato or wholegrain brown rice (not white).

Choose from the salads shown on pages 175–8. *Do not* use the dressings shown, as these contain dairy produce. The following dressing is made totally from natural ingredients:

Juice of ½ lemon
Juice of 1 orange
A tiny sprinkle of powdered ginger
Black pepper
2 tsp extra virgin olive oil
Fresh parsley or chopped fresh mint to taste

Mix all the ingredients together in a bowl. I use 50/50 orange juice and lemon juice, but you can adjust the amounts according to your own personal taste. Keep in the fridge in a sealed container (preferably dark), but do not use after 24 hours.

Drink

Throughout the day, drink as much water as possible to help your body flush out any toxins that are released. *Do not* drink tea, coffee or any canned drinks. Herbal teas are fine. Fruit juice diluted with water is fine. You can also dilute fresh fruit juice with hot water, which is really nice and very calming for your digestive system. I use 50/50 juice to water, but you can adjust this a little if you prefer a slightly stronger or weaker taste.

Snacks

You may find that you feel quite hungry at first. This is quite normal. It is because your body is expecting its usual food and is responding out of habit. If you want to snack, then any raw vegetable, such as celery, carrots or raw peppers, is fine. Fruit is also fine, but try to avoid too much citrus fruit. Don't limit yourself – if you want something, do have vegetables or fruit. There is nothing to be gained by starving yourself – the idea is to give your body a rest from processed food, not from food altogether!

Part 3: Get Moving!

Chapter 7

Exercise

If you really want to tone up, lose weight and change shape, exercise is crucial.

Exercise means different things to different people. For some it means going for a walk, for others it means running a marathon. One of these examples is enough to promote good health and the other is excessive for most people (including me!) Guess which is which?!

The amount of exercise you do must reflect what you want to achieve, that is, the state of health you would like to be in or the weight you would like to be. If your normal daily requirements for energy don't require you to be fit enough to run a marathon, then why train as if you were going to run one?

NO PAIN, NO GAIN?

Many people when they begin an exercise programme for the first time make the mistake of thinking that they have to work really hard in order to achieve anything. This is quite wrong. The most important step you will ever take in terms of exercise is the one that takes you from doing nothing to doing something, whatever that something is. In fact, research published over recent years shows quite clearly that even regular walks at a pace fast enough to raise your heart rate to above its normal level without leaving you feeling over challenged are enough to initiate changes and benefits to your health. So what are you waiting for?

The best possible way to start any exercise programme is to choose a form of exercise that you enjoy doing, otherwise you won't stick to it. If you haven't exercised before, start nice and gently, with the 'easy does it' approach. Remember, anything is better than nothing and everyone can do *something*. Your ideal programme will contain exercises you enjoy doing without leaving you feeling exhausted.

If you exercise regularly, not only will it help you to lose weight, tone up and change shape, but you will be making your heart stronger, improving your muscle tone, helping your body to build strong healthy bones and reducing your risk of suffering from osteoporosis. People who are active not only look better, but they feel better. They are better able to cope with the stress and strain of everyday life, and are more likely to recover quickly from illness. With regular exercise, you will notice a difference within two or three weeks, or less. You will discover energy reserves you didn't even know you had. And you can achieve all of these benefits without any pain or discomfort. You may even enjoy yourself! You will certainly enjoy how you start to feel.

Scientists have been looking at the benefits of different types of exercise programmes for several years and I have used some of that valuable information to design the exercise programme in this chapter. However, because we are all different, you may need to adapt how much you do and how long you do it for. But if you follow the guidelines I give you, you can be assured that your exercise programme will be both safe and effective.

WHICH EXERCISE BURNS THE MOST CALORIES?

People often say to me, 'I know exercise burns calories, but which exercises burn the most?' The answer isn't as simple as you might expect. It generally follows that the harder you work, the more calories you burn. However the body has two sources of fuel to choose from to give us the energy we need to exercise and it has to decide which is the more efficient for the job.

Sugar for Energy

If you are working very hard, the majority of calories you burn will come from glucose. As already explained, this comes from carbohydrate foods that have been broken down into tiny glucose molecules. We all have glucose in our blood (blood sugar) and also store small amounts in our muscles (glycogen). This can be burnt quite effectively to give our muscles the power to contract, but the supplies are limited. Once they have been used up, our muscles feel very heavy and tired and we have to rest until our stores can be replenished. This kind of exercise is called 'anaerobic', which simply means that we are not using oxygen to help us burn the glycogen. We are not burning fat either.

Fat is Best

If you undertake a more moderate programme, for example brisk walking or cycling at a moderate pace, then your body has more time to take the fat out of your fat cells and release it into the blood where it can be transported to the working muscles which can then break it down and use it for energy. This type of exercise is called 'aerobic'. This simply means that you are using oxygen to help you burn the fat.

Although you might not burn as many calories in total if you compare brisk walking to running, if you are a newcomer to exercise or want to lose weight, this is a good form of exercise, as most of the calories you burn will come from fat.

STRENGTHEN YOUR HEART

Another advantage of aerobic exercise is that it strengthens the heart and the circulation system. The heart becomes slightly larger and stronger. This reduces your risk of suffering from heart disease. People who take regular aerobic exercise usually have a lower resting heart rate and lower blood pressure. Some research has indicated that if you have eaten a diet high in saturated fat and your arteries have begun to clog up with fatty deposits, exercise can actually help to break these down and clear the arteries.

If you don't exercise, you lose the elasticity in your lungs and the amount of oxygen you can take in and use (VO_2 max) is reduced. This means you become out of breath very quickly. Respiratory muscles are like any other muscles – if they are not challenged, they become weaker and smaller. Luckily, like other muscles, they can be trained to become stronger and more efficient again.

Exercise also decreases the amount of cholesterol in the blood, making you less prone to blood clots which can cause heart attacks or strokes.

LET'S LOSE WEIGHT!

If you want to lose weight, you should include some kind of aerobic activity, sustained for between 10 to 30 minutes depending on your fitness level, two or three times a week. You should also include some toning exercises for your muscles. That way you will be increasing your muscle tone, which means that your muscles will be able to burn more calories on a daily basis, even when you are not exercising.

MUSCLES BURN FAT

The amount of calories we require each day in order to remain alive is dependent on the amount of muscle tissue we have. On average, every pound (0.4 kg) of muscle tissue requires approximately 40 calories per day.

As mentioned earlier, if you don't exercise and your muscles become smaller and weaker, you will probably replace the lost muscle tissue with body fat, as the body has to store the excess calories that you cannot now burn. Although your weight may not change very much on the scales, as muscle weight lost is replaced with fat weight gained, clothes will become tighter and you will see your skin becoming very fleshy. You look fatter because you *are* fatter.

The only way to reduce this body fat is to control what you eat and to burn off the excess. You cannot do this overnight, but you can replace lost muscle tissue quite quickly. Although it may have taken you several years to lose it, you can replace it within several months.

BODY WEIGHT

Your body weight can be divided up into two areas (apart from the water content): the first is called lean body mass (LBM); the second is called fat. LBM refers to all your muscles, the weight of your bones (remember bones are incredibly light, so you can't blame 'having a heavy frame' for your weight) and your internal organs. What's left when you take all of this away is fat.

As explained on pages 67–75, fat is essential and serves many functions. When you are on a weight loss programme, we are aiming not just to lose weight, but to lose excess fat weight. This means you should aim to change your body composition, not just to lose weight on the scales regardless of whether you are losing fat, muscle or water. If you want to tone up, lose weight and change shape, you need to reduce your body fat levels. It's as simple as that! This programme will show you how.

You don't have to be a scientist to appreciate the benefits of exercise – once you have started a regular exercise programme you will be the best judge of the benefits, as you will see and feel them personally!

A GENTLE START

When choosing your exercise programme, you don't have to start with something new that you have never done before. For example, you don't have to launch yourself into your nearest aerobics class if you don't feel ready. Try starting by walking a mile (1.6 km) at a comfortable pace, but faster than you would normally walk, so that you start to sweat and you can feel that your heart rate has increased. If you are quite comfortable at this level, increase the distance by half a mile. Ideally you want to build up to walking for 30 minutes at this pace. This should be followed by the cool down stretches shown on pages 115–18. If five minutes is sufficient for you to begin with, start with that and increase the time as you feel comfortable and able to do so.

The golden rule is: 'Anything is better than nothing!' As your confidence and your fitness levels increase and you can walk briskly for 30 minutes without feeling exhausted, then you are probably ready to try a fitness video (The *Fat to Flat* workout is now available on video.) or an aerobics class, if you want to. If you are happier walking, then walk a little faster, take longer strides and use as many muscles as you can as you stride along. This is called 'power walking' and is a great form of fat-burning exercise.

Other aerobic activities you could try include:

badminton
tennis
bicycling
dancing

swimming
skipping
stationary cycles
rowing machines
stepping machines

TONE UP

Toning exercises are also very beneficial, not just for losing weight but also for maintaining healthy muscles and bones to protect your joints and improve your posture.

As with aerobic exercise, you don't have to work very hard to see improvements. You are not training for a marathon or for a weight-lifting contest! The aim is to ensure that your body is functioning as well as it possibly can, not only to help you burn more calories and lose weight, but also to enjoy the good health that you are entitled to.

Remember, toning exercises help to burn calories, but they also increase the amount of muscle you have on your body, which in turn helps you to burn even more calories, all the time, even when you are not exercising.

KEEP IT UP

When you achieve good muscle tone, your body will look better and your weight loss will be more noticeable. Exercise also stimulates the digestive system and helps to keep the bowels regular; in other words, it is a natural laxative. This is also very important if you want to lose weight, as explained earlier.

When you exercise, you are doing something positive for your body. But you cannot store the benefits you will achieve. If you stop exercising, then all the muscle tissue that you have built will start to shrink again. You will be burning fewer calories and will probably regain the weight you have lost. So you need to keep it up.

One of the most important aspects of staying motivated is to remind yourself *why* you are exercising. On the days when you feel as though you can't be bothered, ask yourself whether or not you want to continue to lose weight. If the answer is yes, then you should make sure you exercise that day, because if you start to skip a session here and there, it will soon increase to the point where you are constantly putting it off until tomorrow – and we all know tomorrow never comes!

If you usually go walking, for example, but it's cold or raining and you really don't fancy going outside, try something else instead. Either do the toning exercises at home or try something indoors, swimming for example, just make sure you do *something*. Constantly remind yourself that every time you exercise you are one step closer to achieving and maintaining your goal. Make exercise a habit, a *positive habit*.

YOUR EXERCISE PROGRAMME

AEROBIC EXERCISE

Choose one of the examples on page 108 for your aerobic work-out. You should aim to do this for up to

30 minutes, two to three times per week. You can vary the activity – for example, if it is a lovely day try power walking and if it is raining, get your favourite aerobic exercise video out and do that instead. It doesn't matter what the activity is, if it is causing your heart to work faster to pump more oxygen around the body, then it is aerobic.

If you are a newcomer to exercise or haven't exercised for many years, then you should start gently. Five or ten minutes may be enough for you initially. You will find that you can quickly increase the amount of time you can manage if you work out in this way two or three times per week.

The body burns more fat after about 10 minutes, so the sooner you can break this barrier the better. However, you should always feel comfortable, never overtired or gasping for breath. Everyone has their own individual aerobic capability, so listen to your body.

I find the best way to monitor the intensity level is to use the Perceived Rate of Exertion scale (below). Simply compare how you feel to the number and explanation on the scale. Make sure you do not go above number seven, but try to get over number four:

Level 1. No effort
Level 2. Slight effort
Level 3. Effort required
Level 4. Rate of breathing starting to increase
Level 5. Slightly breathless, starting to perspire
Level 6. Breathless but comfortable, perspiring freely
Level 7. More breathless, able to speak short sentences

Level 8. More breathless, only able to speak a few words
Level 9. Very breathless, unable to speak, feeling tired
Level 10. Very breathless, heavy legs, unable to continue

THE WARM UP

You will need to warm up and stretch before you begin your aerobic work-out. Spend about five minutes doing the following exercises:

Pulse Raising and Mobility

March on the Spot
Start with small marches and then start to lift the knees higher and move the arms more.

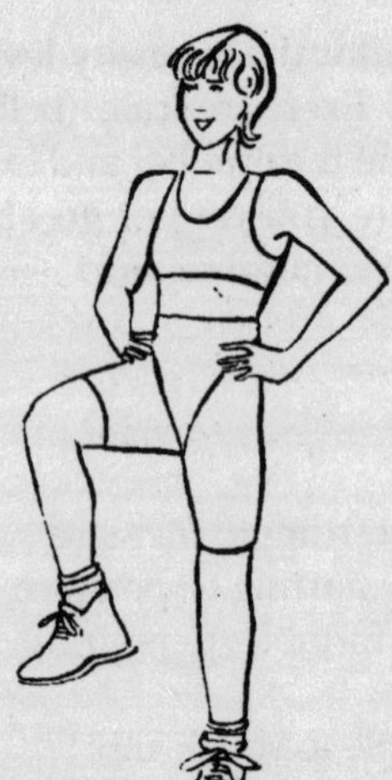

Knee Lifts
Keeping the back nice and tall and the shoulders back, raise alternate knees to approximately hip height.

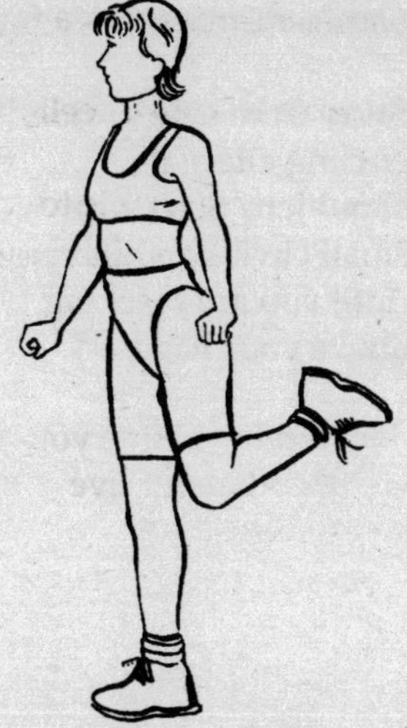

Hamstring Curls
Step from side to side, kicking your bottom with alternate heels.

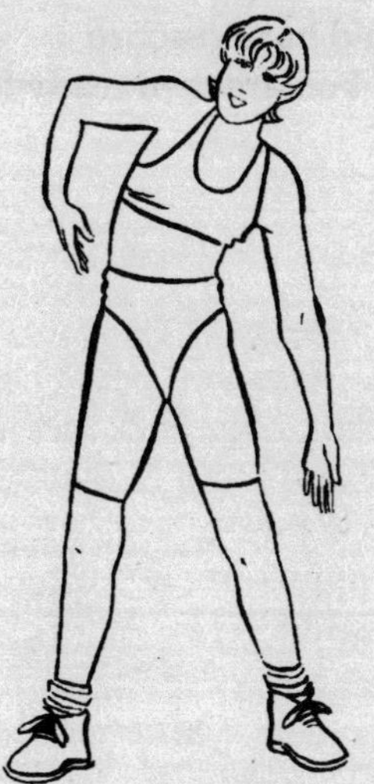

Side Bends
Stand with your feet apart, keep your knees soft and your hips still, and gently reach down from side to side.

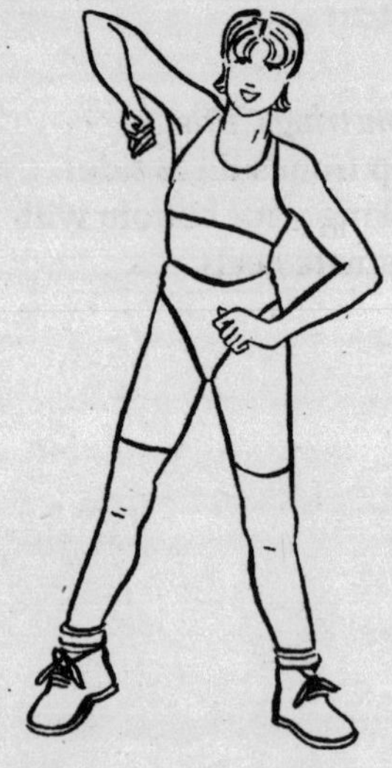

Shoulder Circles

Sway from side to side, circling alternate shoulders. Start with small circles and increase until you are reaching above your head.

After these exercises, you should have reached number four on the PRE scale. You are then ready to do the stretches.

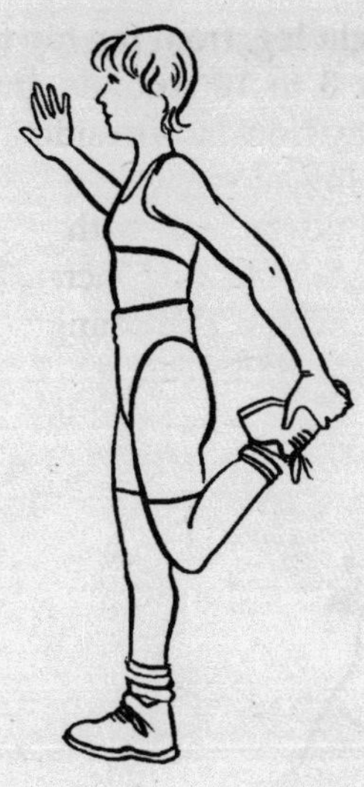

Stretches

Quads (front of thigh)
Using a wall for balance, place one foot in your hand and ease the leg back slowly until the knee is behind the hip. Keep the hips square, pull your tummy in to support your back and tilt the pelvis under. You should feel the stretch across the front of the hip and down the front of the thigh. Hold for 8 to 10 seconds and repeat with the other leg.

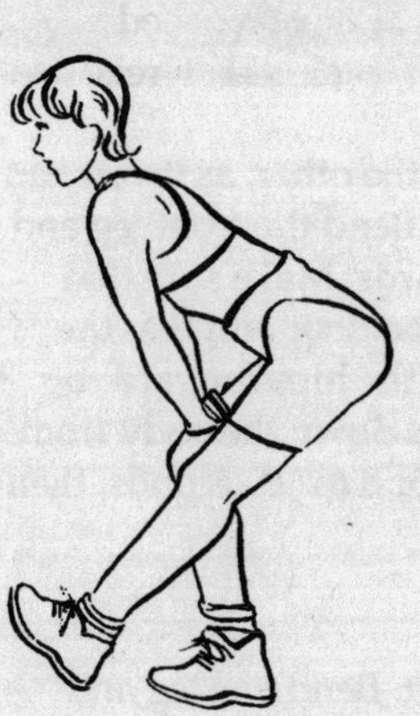

Hamstrings (back of thigh)
Stand with one foot in front of the other, as if you had taken a generous stride forwards, and transfer all of your weight to your back leg. Bending the leg, sit down into the stretch. Support your body weight with both hands on the thigh of the bent leg and tilt the pelvis so that the base of your spine is towards the ceiling. Keep the hips square. You should feel

this down the back of the straight leg, from the hip to just below the knee. Hold for 8 to 10 seconds and repeat with the other leg.

Gastrocnemius (calf)

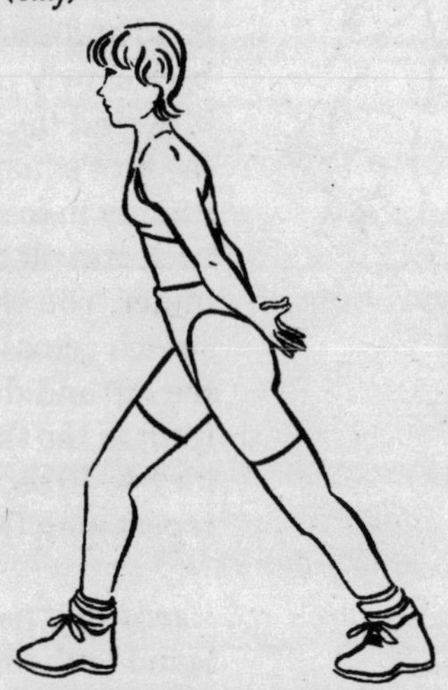

Stand with one foot in front of the other, as if you had taken a generous stride ahead. Bend the front leg and transfer the body weight forwards. Make sure that the heel of the back foot is on the floor and that the toes are facing forwards. Press the hips forward to ensure that a diagonal line runs down the body from your head to your toes. Hold for 8 to 10 seconds, then repeat with the other leg.

Adductors (inner thigh)
Stand with your feet wide apart. Bend one leg and transfer the body weight over to this leg. Make sure that your knee does not go over the line of your toe.

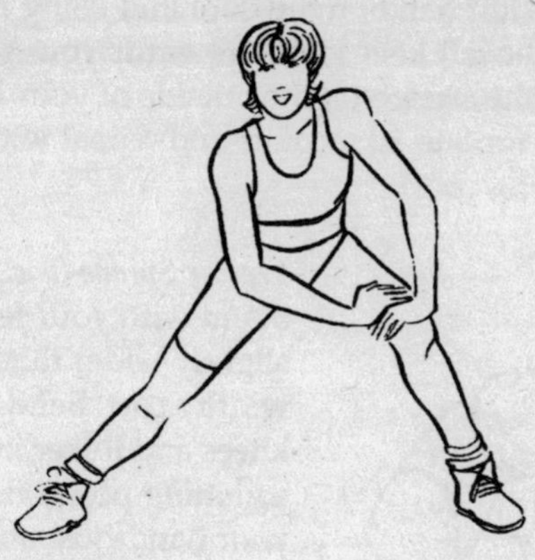

You should be able to see your foot. If not, your feet are too close together. Keep the hips square to the front. You should feel this on the inside of the thigh on the straight leg. Hold for 8 to 10 seconds and repeat with the other leg.

Abductors (outside thigh)

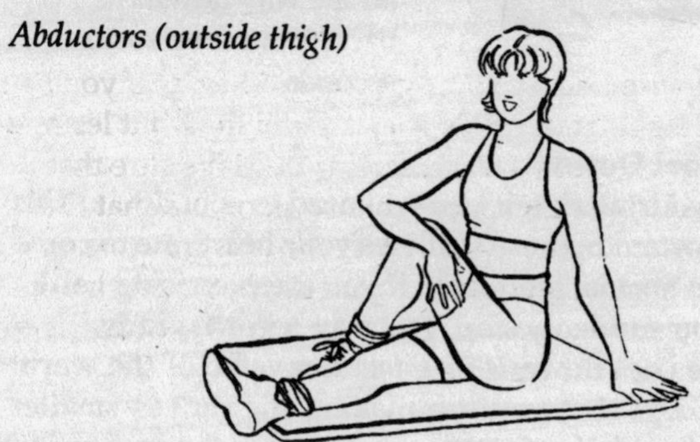

Sit on the floor with your right leg straight in front of you. Bend the left knee and cross it over the right leg.

Keeping the left hand on the floor and using the right hand, pull the left knee gently towards you. You should feel the stretch on the outside of your left thigh. Hold for 8 to 10 seconds and repeat with the other leg.

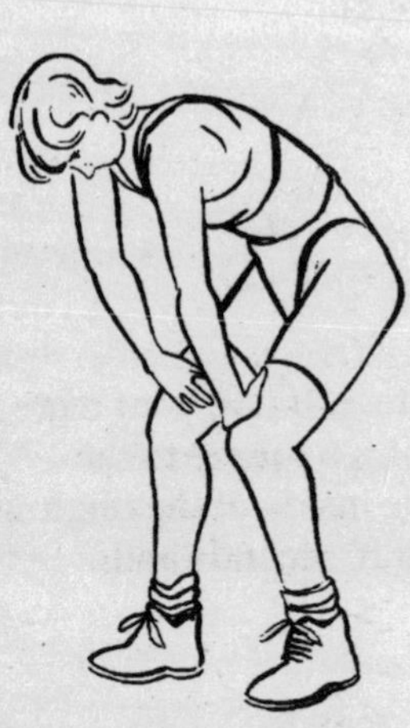

Erector Spinae (back)
Stand with your feet slightly wider than hip width apart. Bend the knees and lower into a squatting position. Place your hands just above your knees and support your body weight on your arms. Pull the tummy in and tuck your head and pelvis under to arch the spine. You should feel this all the way down the back. Hold for 8 to 10 seconds.

The Cool Down

After your work-out you will need to cool down. This is important because it allows your heart rate to come back to normal gradually. If you are exercising hard and you suddenly stop, you may become giddy.

The cool down is in effect a reverse of the warm up, except that you are making the moves smaller instead of bigger. Start by marching on the spot, using your arms and lifting your knees, and gradually reduce the intensity by lowering the arms and the legs. This may take three or four minutes, depending on how hard you have been working and how long you have been working for.

After you have cooled down you should be able to feel that your heart rate has returned to a more normal level. If not, you should keep moving for a while until it does. Once you feel it has come down, repeat the stretches as before.

BODY SHAPING EXERCISES

Choose the area that you would most like to work on. If you are a rounded shape and want to flatten your tummy, you will find lots of different exercises to firm up the abdominal muscles. If you are more of a pear shape, you will find lots of exercises for the hips and thighs. There is also a section to improve posture. You will find this particularly beneficial if you are tall or if you have to bend over a lot. People who work at a desk, for example, often become very round shouldered as back muscles weaken. If you correct this, then your whole posture and appearance improves. I have also included a few more general exercises which can include if you wish to. In each case I have explained the muscles which you will be working and how the exercise will improve your overall shape.

Ideally you should do your aerobic work-out three times per week and your toning exercises three times per week. As this section will only take you about 10 minutes, you may find you are able to do it more often. If you wish to combine it with your aerobic work and do both together, that's fine.

WARMING UP

Before any of the body shaping exercises, you will need to do some warming up exercises for the muscles you are going to work. These exercises are shown at the beginning of each section.

After you have finished the warm up, complete the stretches shown on page 115. This will help to prevent the muscles feeling tight after your work-out.

APPLE SHAPE

If you are an apple shape, your target area is your abdominal muscles. Many people think that the only abdominal exercise you need to do is the traditional abdominal curl, or sit up. This is very wrong. The area between the ribs and the pelvic girdle is completely unprotected by the skeleton, yet it contains some of the most vital internal organs. To make up for this lack of bone, we have several layers of muscle to hold everything in place and protect us. These are what you need to work on!

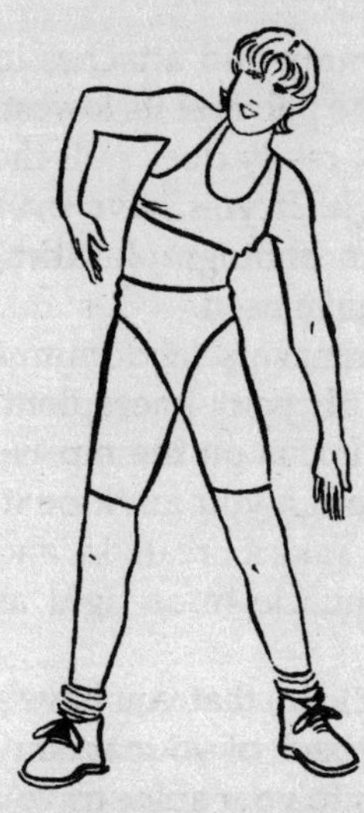

Warm Up

Side Bends
Stand with your feet hip width apart. Keeping the hips square to the front, lean slowly down to each side, as far as is comfortable.

Body Shaping Exercises

Controlled Press: Transverse Abdominus

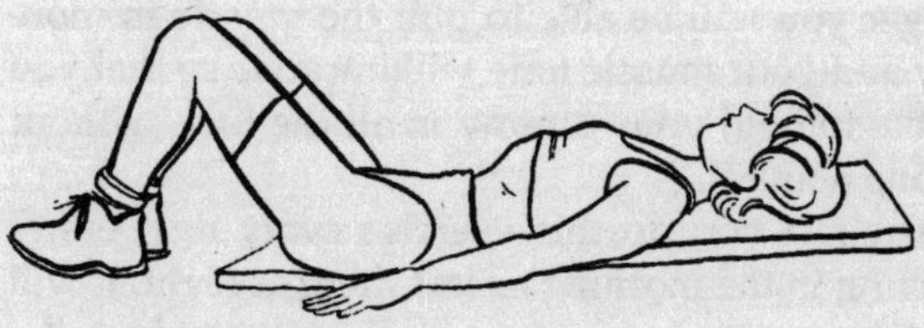

The most important abdominal muscle to exercise if you want to achieve a flatter tummy is the transverse abdominus. This muscle wraps around us like a huge belt. It starts one side of the spine, goes around the front and then back to the other side of the spine. It opens up at the front of the tummy and attaches to the ribs at its highest point and the pelvis at its lowest. It is a huge sheet of muscle that really does pull the tummy in if it is strong enough. If you have ever pulled your tummy in to have a photograph taken, then this is the muscle you will have used.

The best way to work your transverse abdominus muscle is to lie on the floor with your knees bent. Relax your arms by your side. Focus on the muscle that you are going to work, although you can't see it, picture where it is in your mind. Take a breath in, and as you breathe out, pull this muscle in as tight as you can.

Imagine, as you pull the muscle in, that you have a piece of blu-tack attached to the back of your tummy button and you want to stick it onto your spine as you press down. Hold for two seconds and release.

Repeat this as many times as you can until you can really feel the muscle has been working. There is almost no movement in the exercise, although you may feel the pelvis roll slightly. As the muscle gets stronger you will be able to pull the muscle in more easily and your muscle tone will improve so that you are able to hold your tummy in all the time without thinking about it.

I suggest you do this exercise every day, either first thing in the morning or last thing at night. It will only take a couple of minutes, but may reduce the size of your tummy by several inches – well worth the effort!

All of the other exercises in this section should be completed at the same time as doing the controlled press. In other words, there's no point in doing an abdominal curl without first controlling this muscle.

Abdominal Curl: Rectus Abdominus

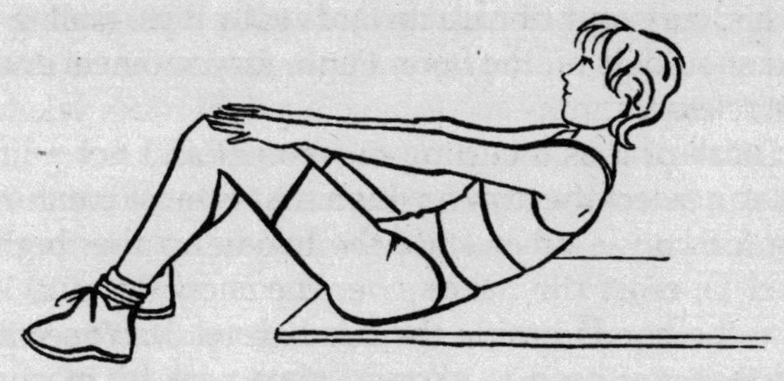

Level 1

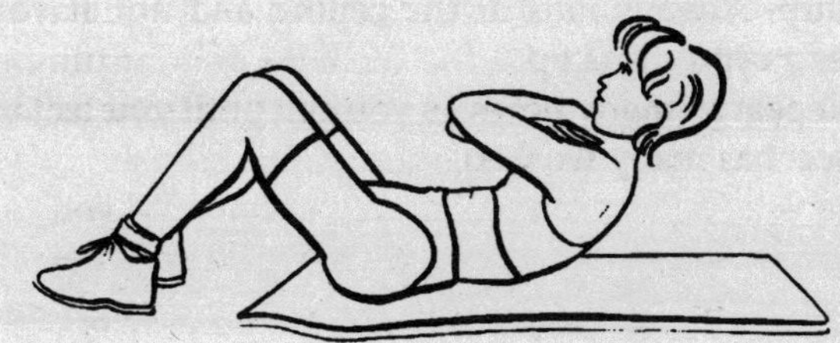

Level 2

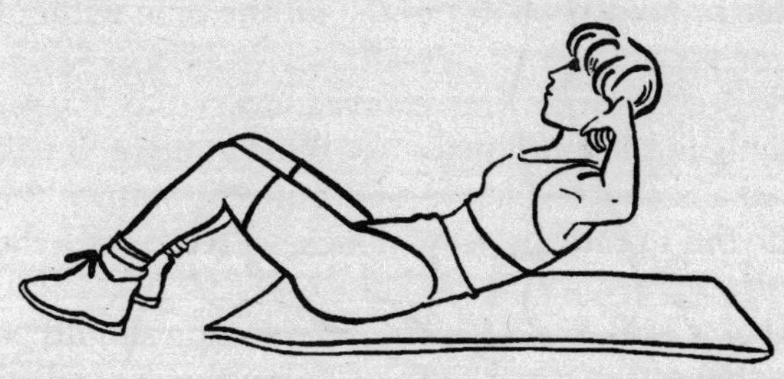

Level 3

Lie on your back with your knees bent. Press your tummy down into the floor (controlled press). As you do this, curl your ribs up towards your hips, raising your shoulders off the floor. Pause for a moment and then release.

Think of it as a curling movement and not a lift. You can select the arm position that is most comfortable for you – either slide the hands up the thighs (level 1), cross the hands over the chest (level 2) or place the hands beside the head (level 3). You may find that you need to support your neck by placing one or both hands on the back of your neck and allowing your head to rest on your forearm as your curl up. Always look at the ceiling and not at your knees as you come up.

Repeat as many times as you can until you feel the muscle has really worked.

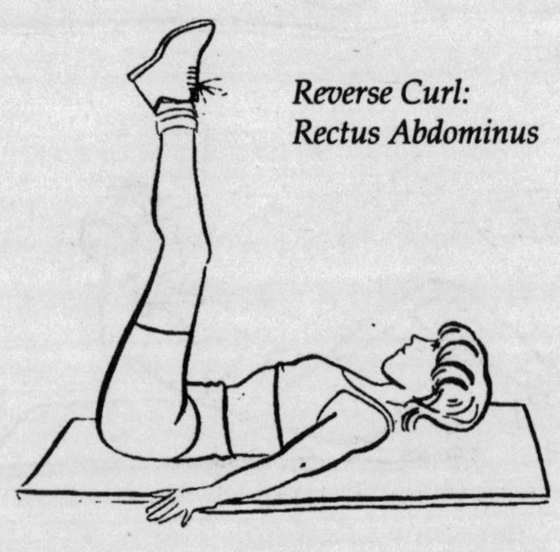

Reverse Curl: Rectus Abdominus

This exercise is particularly beneficial for the lower part of the abdominal muscles. It requires a certain amount of control and really is an extension of the controlled press.

Lie on your back and bring your knees into your chest. Slightly extend the legs. You must make sure that your knees are always over your tummy button. If your legs are further towards the floor your back will arch and you will feel a pull on your lower back. The back should remain flat to the floor at all times. Pull the tummy muscles in and press the tummy down as hard as you can. You may find that you get a slight rocking of the pelvis – this is fine as long as it is because you are using your tummy muscles and not swinging your legs. The technique is exactly the same as the controlled press. Breathe out as you push down.

Repeat this as many times as you can until you feel the muscle has really worked.

Oblique Curl

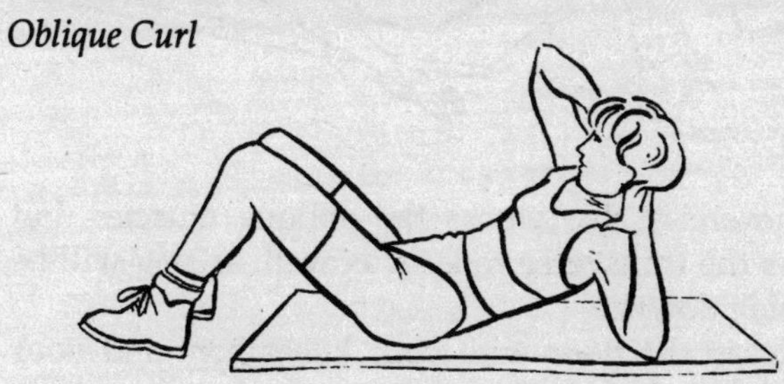

This exercise works the muscles at the side of the waist. They provide extra protection and also enable us to move our spine sidewards. This is very similar to the abdominal curl, except that you turn the trunk slightly as you lift. As with the abdominal curl, you need to do a controlled press as you lift.

Lie on the floor with your feet wider than hip width apart. Keep the hips quite still and press the tummy down. As you do so, lift the ribs and the shoulders off the floor and turn towards your right knee. Your nose should be facing your knee. Keep the chin off the chest. Uncurl and repeat to the other side.

You may find that you need to support your neck in the same way you did with the abdominal curl. Do as many as you can until you feel the muscles have really worked.

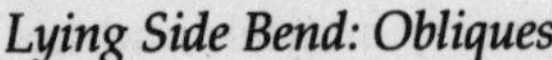

Lying Side Bend: Obliques

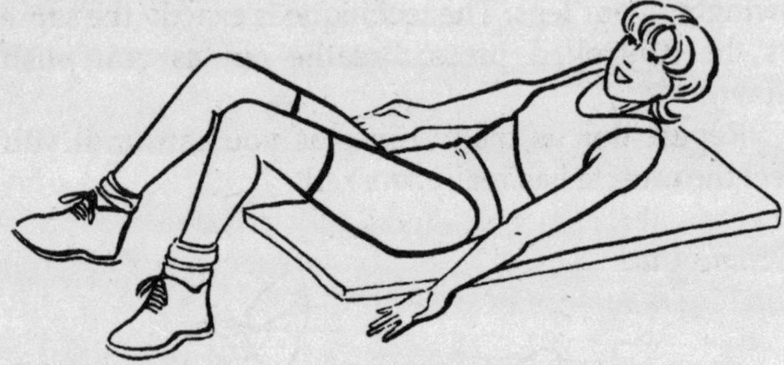

This exercise also works the oblique muscles, but works the transverse muscle as well, as you will be pressing down.

Lie on the floor with your knees bent and your arms by your side. Press the tummy down and very slightly raise your upper back off the floor. Ease your body to the right and reach your right hand down your right thigh. Return to the start position and repeat to the other side.

You may find that you need to support your neck

with your left hand. If so, rest in between each exercise for a moment. As you get stronger you will be able to go from side to side.

You must make sure that you press your tummy down all the time. Make sure you breathe freely – do not hold your breath.

Lying Side Raise: Obliques

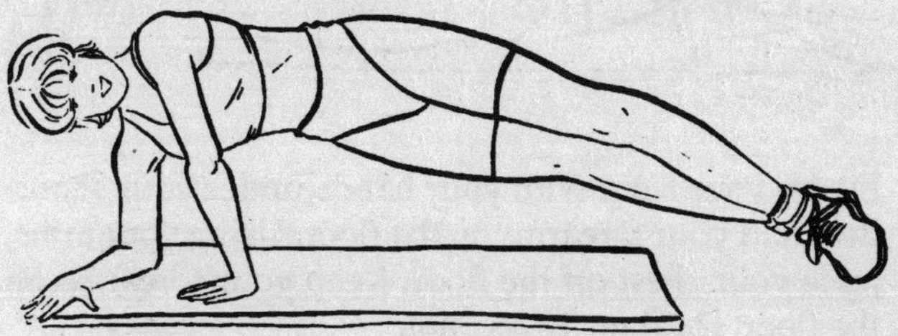

This exercise is quite difficult and you should only include it once you have mastered all the other tummy exercises. If you have a problem with your shoulders, you may wish to leave this one out altogether.

Lie on your right side, supporting your weight on your right elbow. Make sure the elbow is directly beneath the shoulder and the forearm flat on the floor. Place your left foot slightly in front of your right foot so that the sides of both feet are on the floor. You need to pull the muscles in your right side tightly, so that your hips lift off the floor. Only lift as high as is comfortable.

Relax and repeat as many times as you can until you feel the muscles have really worked. Roll over and repeat on the other side.

Stretches

Sphinx

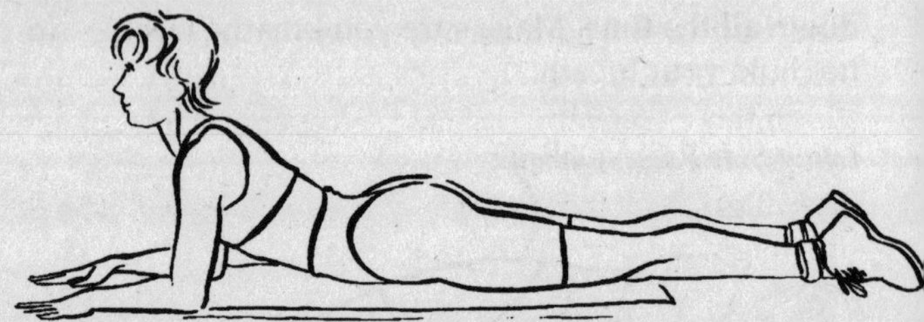

Lie on your front with your hands under your shoulders and your forearms on the floor. Using your arms, raise your chest off the floor. Keep your forearms on the floor. Hold for 10 seconds.

Waist

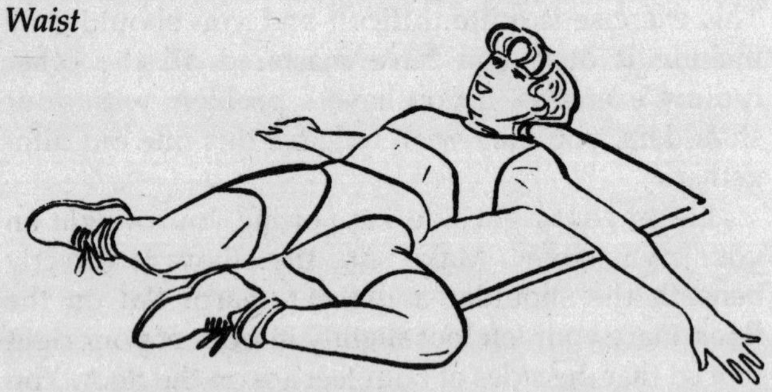

Lie on your back with your knees bent and your feet on the floor. Keeping your feet on the floor, let both knees roll over to one side. Hold for 10 seconds and then repeat to the other side.

PEAR SHAPE

The target areas for this shape are the hips, thighs and buttocks. The muscles we are going to use are the abductors, which are on the outside of the thigh,the adductors, which are on the inside of the thigh, the quadriceps, which are at the front of the thigh, and the gluteals, which are at the side of the thigh and also on the buttocks.

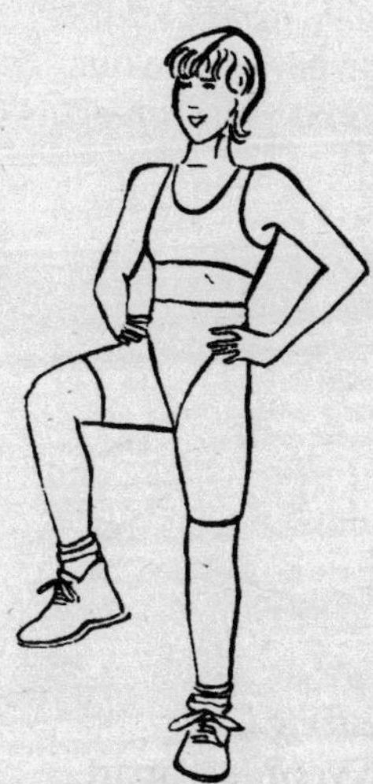

Warm Up

Knee Lift
Standing upright, keep the back tall and raise alternate knees to approximately hip height. Do this about 20 times.

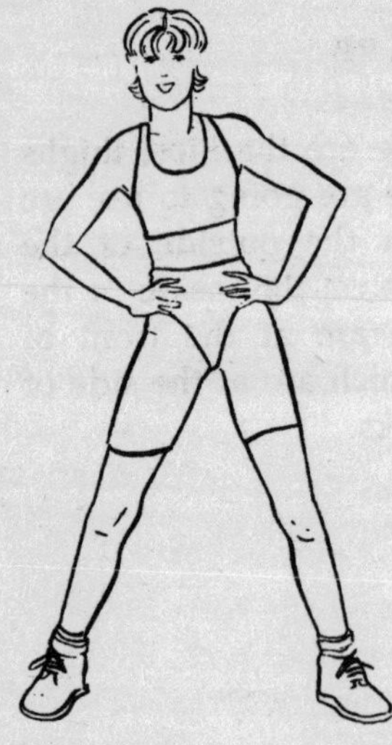

Hip Circles
Stand with your feet hip width apart. Keeping the shoulders still, circle the hips one way and then the other. Repeat 20 times.

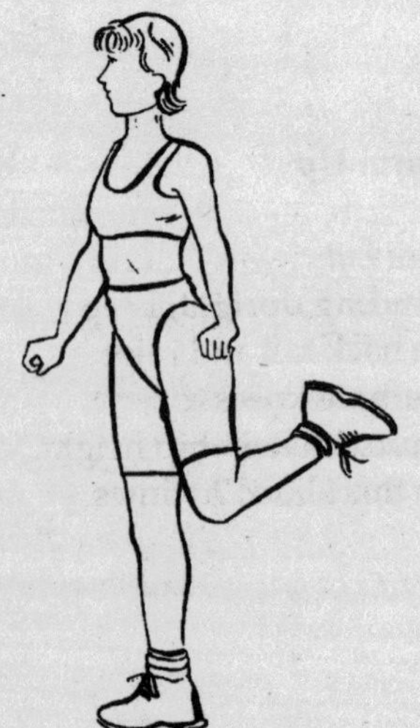

Hamstring Curls
With your feet apart, transfer the weight from one leg to the other and kick your bottom with alternate feet.

Body Shaping Exercises

Standing Squats: Quads and Buttocks

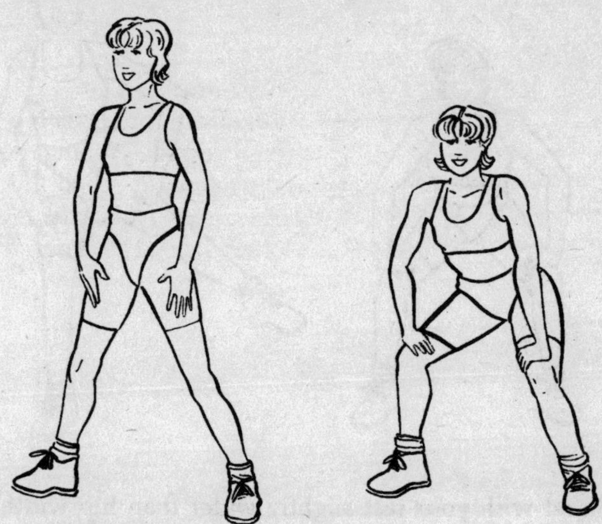

Stand with your feet slightly wider than hip width apart. Turn your toes out slightly so that your knees and toes are facing diagonally outward. Bend your knees and lower your bottom to just above your knees. Place your hands just above your knees to support your weight. As you lower down, push your bottom out slightly behind you. As you straighten the legs to stand up, squeeze the buttocks tightly to push the hips forward.

Repeat as many times as you can until you feel the muscles have really worked.

Squat Raises: Quads, Buttocks and Abductors

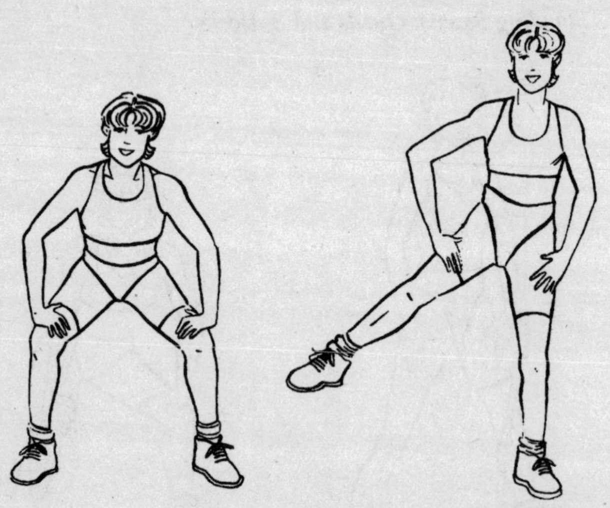

Stand with your feet slightly wider than hip width apart. Turn your toes out slightly so that your knees and toes are facing diagonally outward. Bend your knees and lower your bottom to just above your knees. Place your hands just above your knees to support your weight. As you lower down, push your bottom out slightly behind you.

As you straighten the legs, transfer all the body weight to the left leg and raise the right leg to the side. Make sure you keep the hips square to the front as you raise the leg. Transfer the weight back to both legs and bend into the squat again.

Repeat as many times as possible until you feel the muscles have really worked.

Lunges: Quads and Buttocks

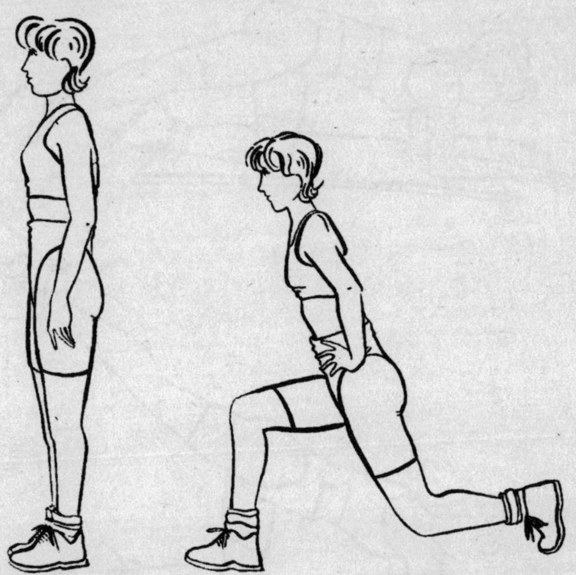

Stand upright with both feet together. Take a large step forward with the right leg and bend the right knee. The knee of the left leg also bends so that the knee goes towards the floor. The closer to the floor the knee is, the harder the exercise is, so you can modify it to make it more comfortable. Push off the front leg (right) and bring the feet together to return to a standing position.

Repeat with the left leg. Do as many as you can until you feel the muscles have really worked.

Gluteal Raises: Buttocks

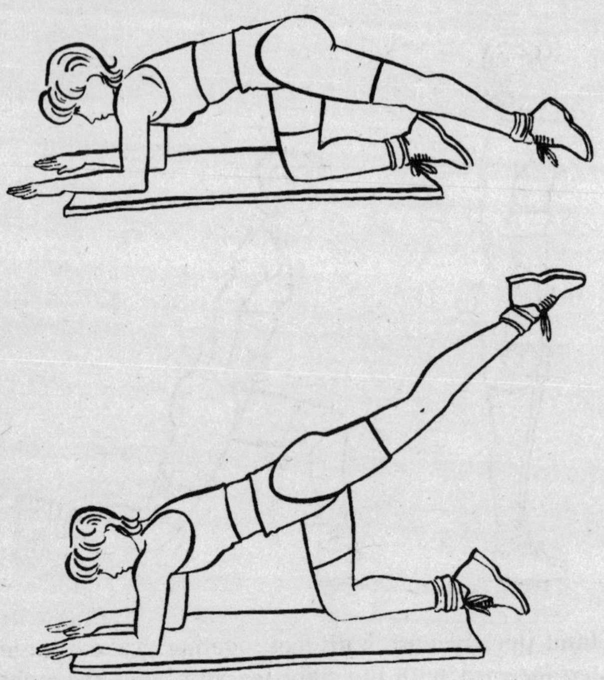

On all fours, place your forearms on the floor. Have your knees directly below your hips and pull the tummy in to support the back. Extend the left leg so that the toe touches the floor. Raise and lower this leg, keeping it as straight as possible, without arching the back.

Repeat as many times as you can until you feel the muscle has really worked, then change legs.

Adductor Raises: Inner Thigh

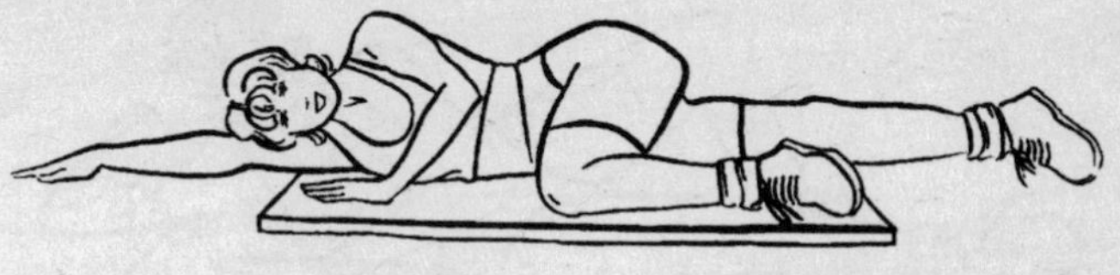

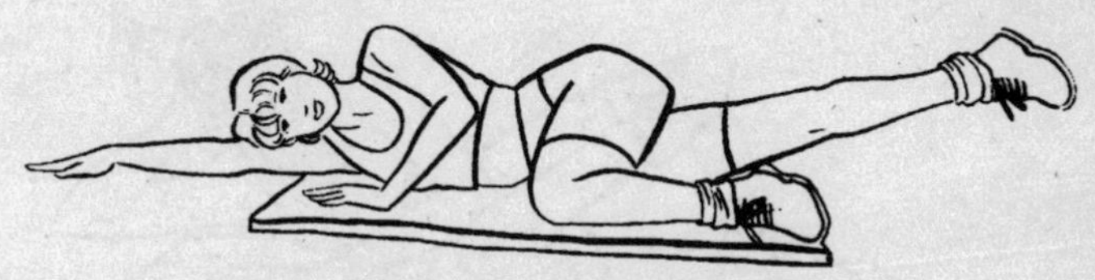

Lie on your right side with your hand supporting your neck or your arm outstretched above you. Place the left knee on the floor in front of you, level with or above the hips. Extend the underneath leg and raise and lower it. As you do so, try to squeeze the muscles on the inside of the thigh to make the exercise more effective. Try not to let the foot touch the floor in between lifts.

Repeat as many times as you can until you feel the muscles have really worked. Roll over and repeat on the other side.

Adductor Raises with Knee Bend: Inner Thigh

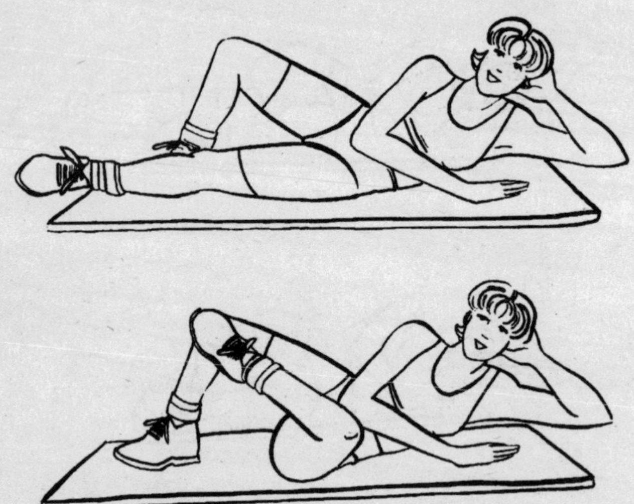

Lie on your left side with your hand supporting your neck or your arm outstretched above you. Bend the right knee and place the right foot behind the left leg, with the knee facing upwards. Keeping the left leg straight, raise the leg, pause, bend the knee so that the left heel touches the right knee, straighten the leg and lower.

Repeat as many times as you can until you feel the muscles have really worked.

Stretches

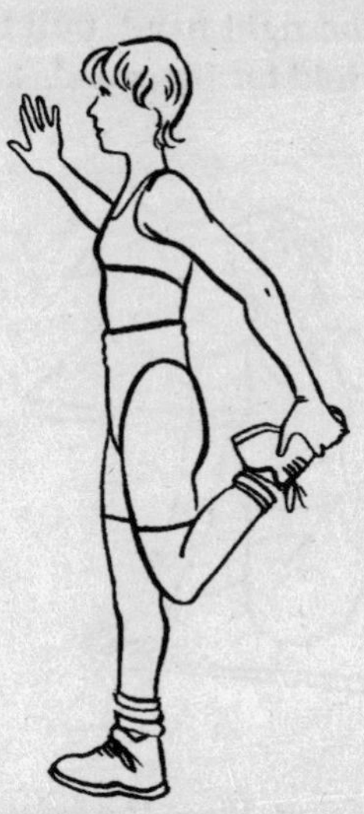

Quads

Lie on your right side with your right arm stretched above your head. Bend the underneath leg to stop you rolling about. Keeping the hips square to the front, bend the left leg and place the foot in the left hand. Squeeze your buttocks to push the hips slightly forward. Hold for 10 seconds. Repeat with the other leg.

Abductors

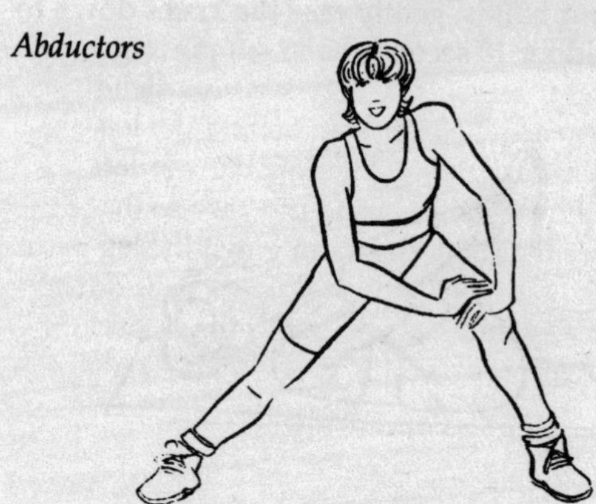

Sit up with the right leg straight in front of you. Bend the left knee and cross it over the right leg. Keep the left hand on the floor. Using the right hand, pull the left knee gently towards you. Hold for 10 seconds and repeat with the other leg.

Adductors

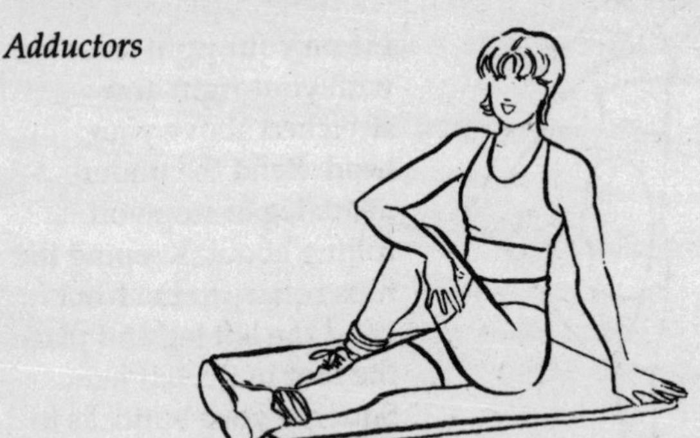

Sit up with your feet in front of you. Place the soles of the feet together and hold the ankles. Using your elbows or your hands, gently ease the knees down to the floor. Hold for 10 seconds.

Gluteals

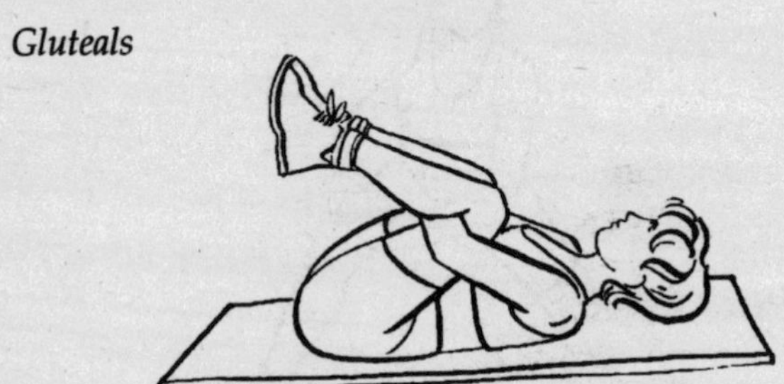

Lie on your back, bring your knees in towards your chest and hold under the thighs. Gently ease the knees towards the chest. Hold for 10 seconds.

POOR POSTURE

Many people have a far better shape than they think, but don't show it, due to bad posture. In particular, taller people often suffer from rounded shoulders because they are continually stooping or bending down. In the same way, if you work at a desk or have any job where you are constantly leaning forwards, you are more likely to suffer from rounded shoulders and weak abdominal and back muscles. Even if you have the best natural shape in the world, if these muscles are weak you will not look your best.

The target areas for the exercises in this section are the upper body, in particular the back muscles. As these muscles get stronger, you will be able to sit or stand more upright. This can have quite a dramatic effect on how you look.

Warm Up Exercises

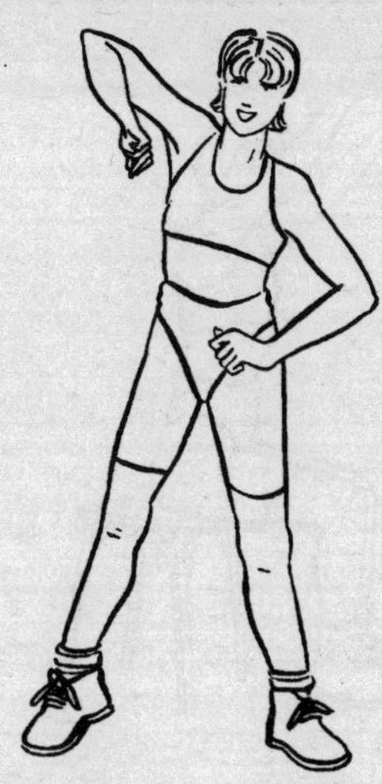

Shoulder Circles
Rotate alternate shoulders backwards. Increase the circle as the shoulders begin to feel looser.

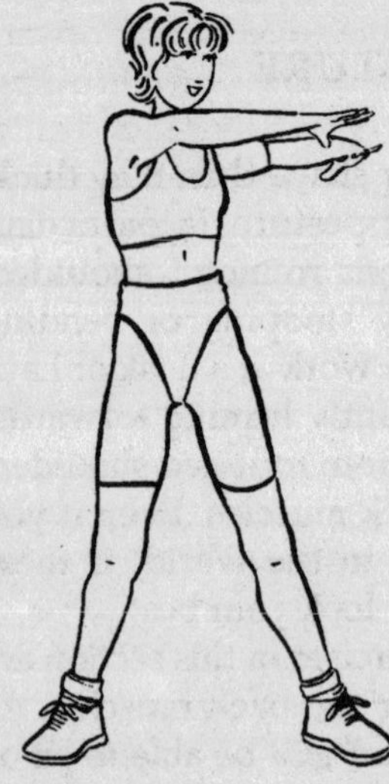

Trunk Twists
Stand with your feet hip width apart. Keep the hips still. Raise the elbows and touch the hands together in front of your chest. Turn slowly to the right and to the left.

Pull Back: Trapezius and Rhomboids

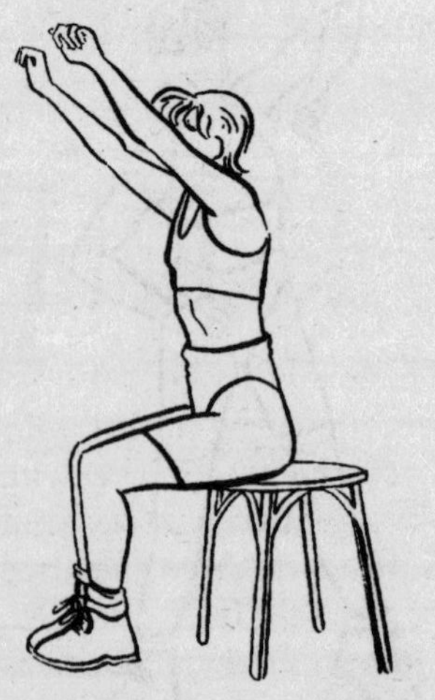

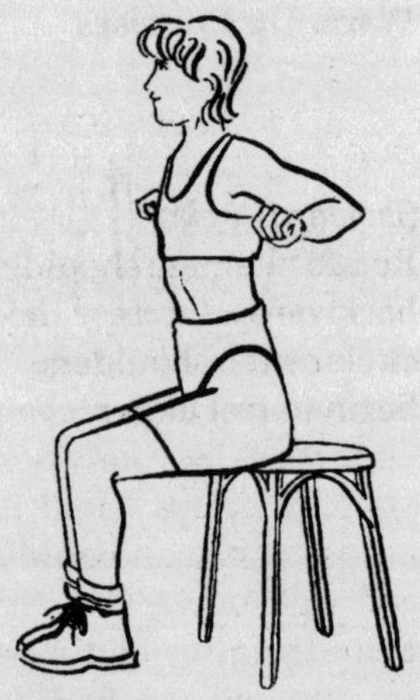

Sit upright in a chair, close to the edge. Reach forward and upwards. Pull your arms back and down in a diagonal line, trying to squeeze your shoulder blades together as you do so. Reach forward and repeat as many times as you can until you feel the muscles have really worked. You can hold light weights, such as tins of food, to make it more difficult, as you grow stronger.

Overhead Press: Deltoids and Triceps

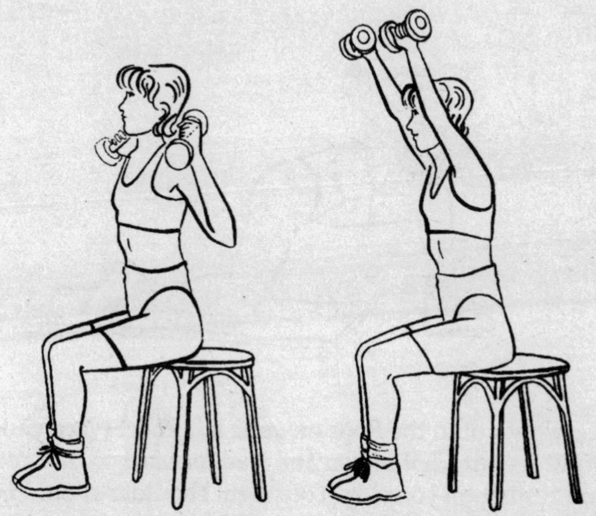

Sitting upright in a chair, bend the arms so that your elbows are by your side and your hands are level with your shoulders. Hold light weights such as a tin of beans or a small bottle of water. Straighten the arms and push upwards so that the arms are fully extended. Bend the arms and repeat. Repeat as many times as you can until you feel the muscles have really worked.

Reverse Fly: Trapezius and Rhomboids

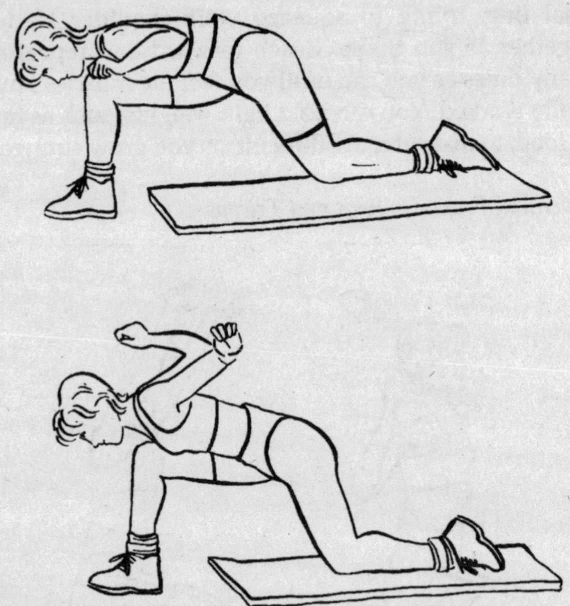

Go down onto the floor on your left knee. Place your right foot in front of you and lean forward so that you are resting on your leg. Your right shoulder should be on your right thigh. You should be able to see your toes clearly. Bend the elbows and take both arms out to the side, so that they are parallel with the floor. From a horizontal position, pull the shoulder blades back and together to raise the arms and then lower.

Repeat as many times as you can until you feel the muscles have really worked.

Shoulder Raises: Deltoids

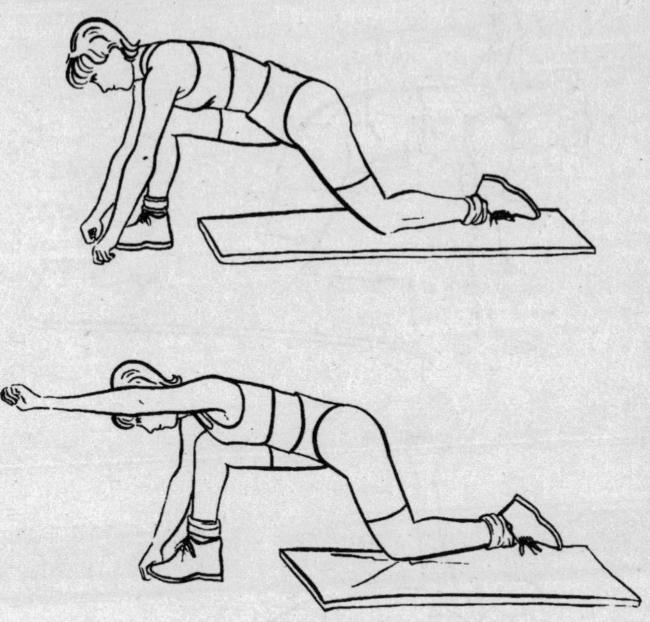

In the same position as before, rest on one knee with both arms touching the floor below your shoulders. Raise alternate arms in front of you to a height approximately level with the shoulders. You may wish to change knees if it becomes uncomfortable.

Lateral Raises: Deltoids

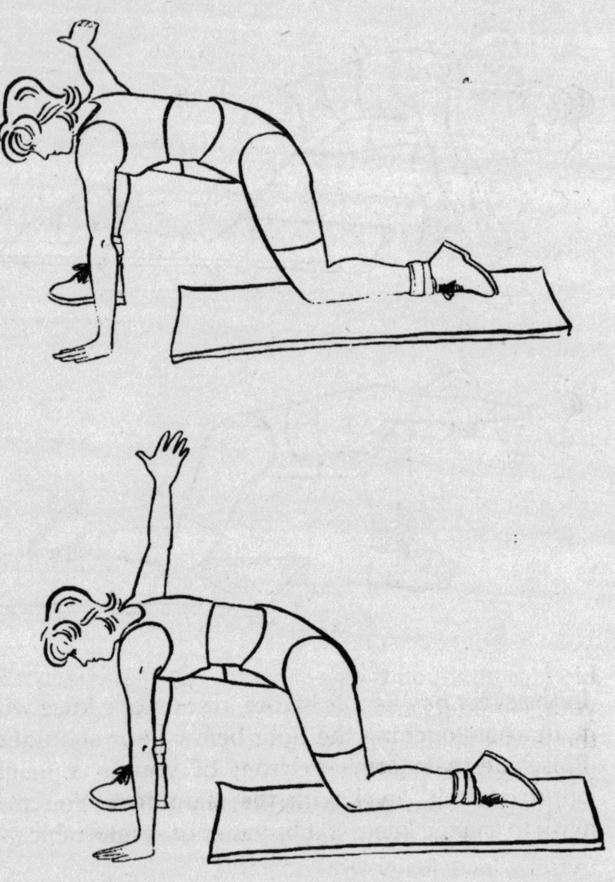

In the same position, raise the right arm to the side so that it is just above the body. Lower and repeat. Do as many as you can until you feel the muscles have really worked. Change legs and work the other arm.

Back Raises: Erector Spinae

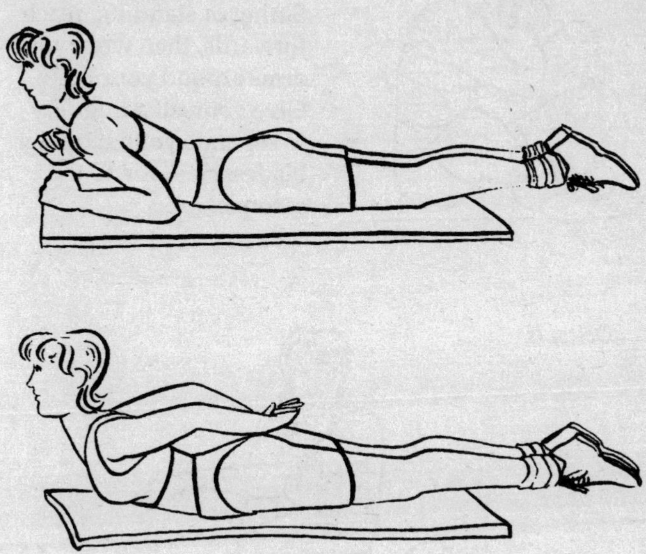

Lie face down on the floor with your hands beneath your shoulders and your forearms on the floor. Keep the hips still and use the muscles in your back to lift your chest off the floor. To make this more difficult, try placing your hands behind your back, on your bottom. Do as many as you can until you feel the muscles have really worked.

Stretches

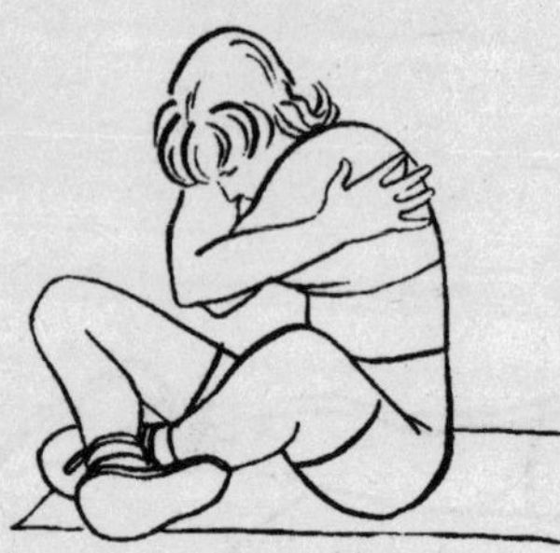

Trapezius and Rhomboids
Sitting or standing, reach forwards, then wrap your arms around your body. Give yourself a hug. Try to separate your shoulder blades. Hold for 10 seconds.

Deltoids

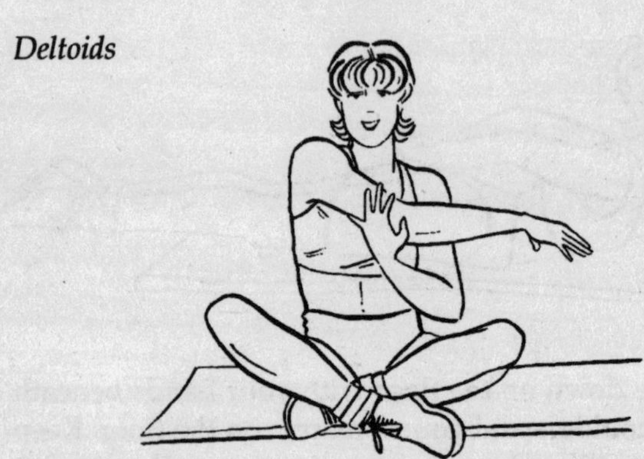

Reach across your chest with your right arm. Using the left hand, gently ease the arm further across. Hold for 10 seconds. Repeat with the other arm.

Erector Spinae

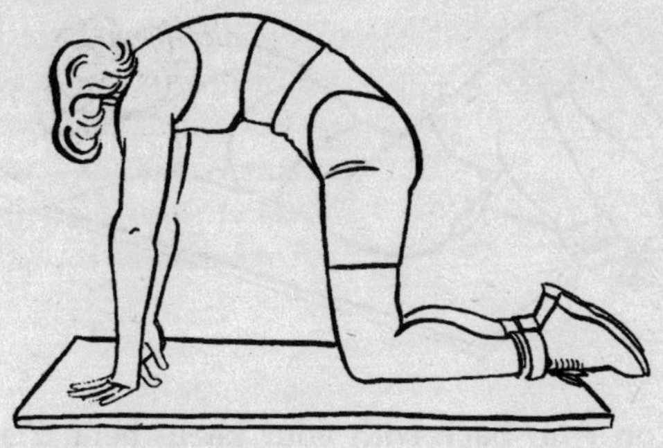

On all fours, arch your back as much as you can. Hold for 10 seconds.

EXERCISES FOR GENERAL TONING

THE BUST

To tone the bust, you need to strengthen the muscles that support it, i.e. the pectorals. These are large muscles that span the chest and are attached to the top of the arm. They are used when you bring your arms towards your chest. The breasts themselves are not made of muscle; they are mostly fat, therefore you cannot directly increase their size by exercising. However, you can lift your bust quite dramatically by working the underlying muscles.

Pec Dec: Pectorals

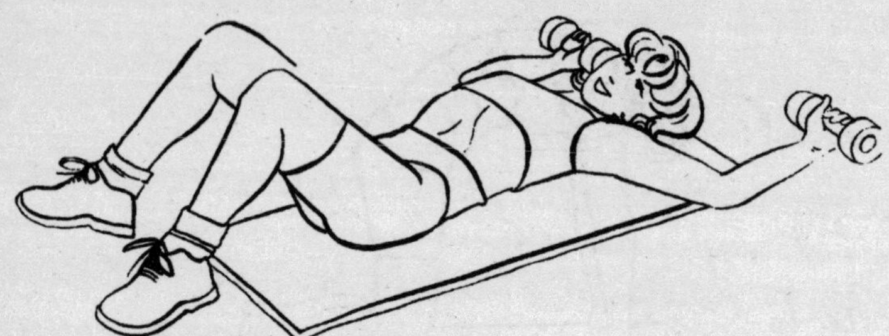

Lie on your back with your knees bent. Place your arms on the floor beside you with elbows bent, in line with your shoulders. Keep the forearm and the hands on the floor. Raise the arms so that you press the forearms and the hands tightly together. Squeeze and take the arms out to the side.

Repeat as many times as you can until you feel the muscles have really worked. To make it more challenging, try holding a can of beans or a small bottle of water.

Box Press: Pectorals

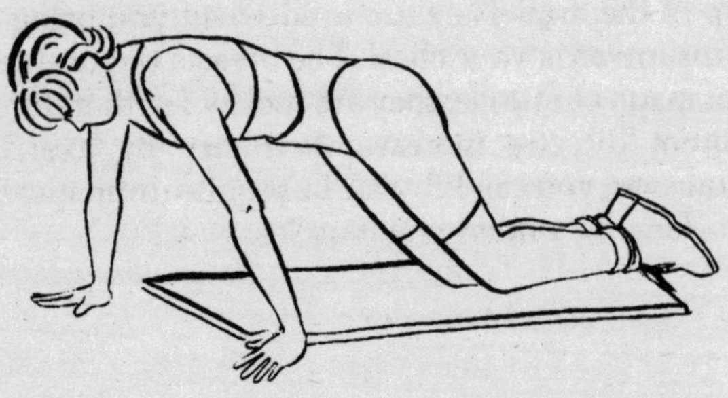

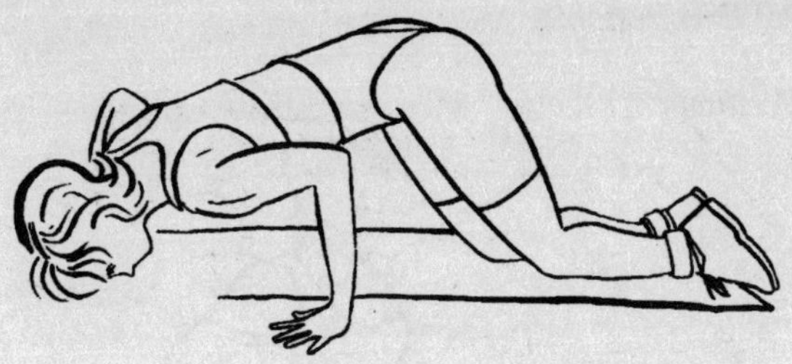

Level 1

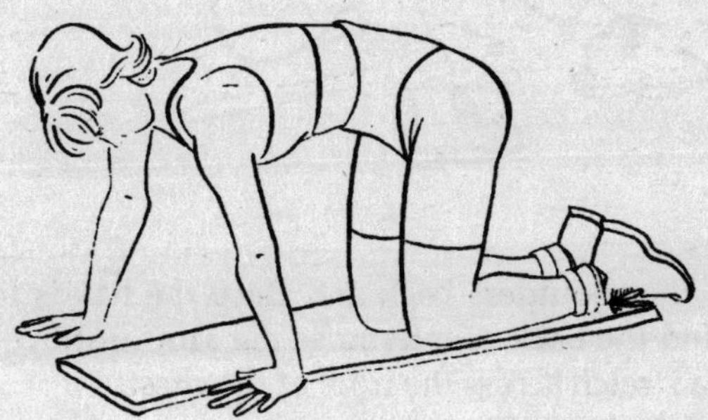

Level 2

On all fours, place your hands wider than shoulder width apart and your knees under your hips, hip width apart. Your chin should be in line with your fingers. Pull your tummy in to support your back and bend your arms slowly, lowering your nose almost to the floor. Straighten your arms and push back up again (level 1). To make this more challenging, take the knees further back (level 2).

Stretch

Pectorals

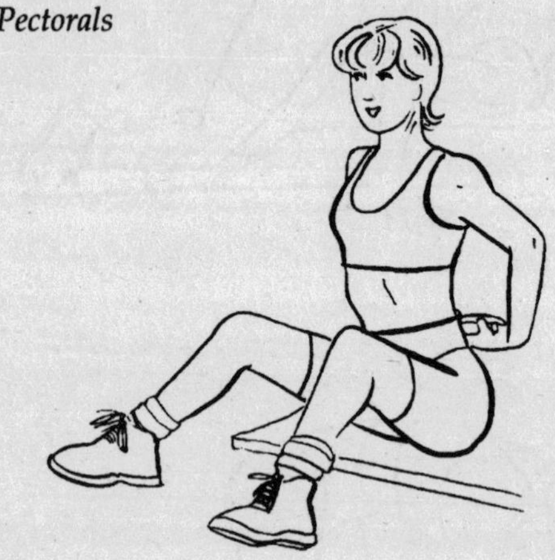

Roll the shoulders back and clasp the hands lightly behind the back. Gently raise the arms until you can feel a stretch across the front of the chest.

FLABBY ARMS

The back of the arms is another area where many people, particularly women, seem to store loose fat. It can make the arms very unsightly and tops with short or no sleeves highlight the problem. To tone up this area, we need to work the tricep muscles at the back of the arm.

Tricep Dip

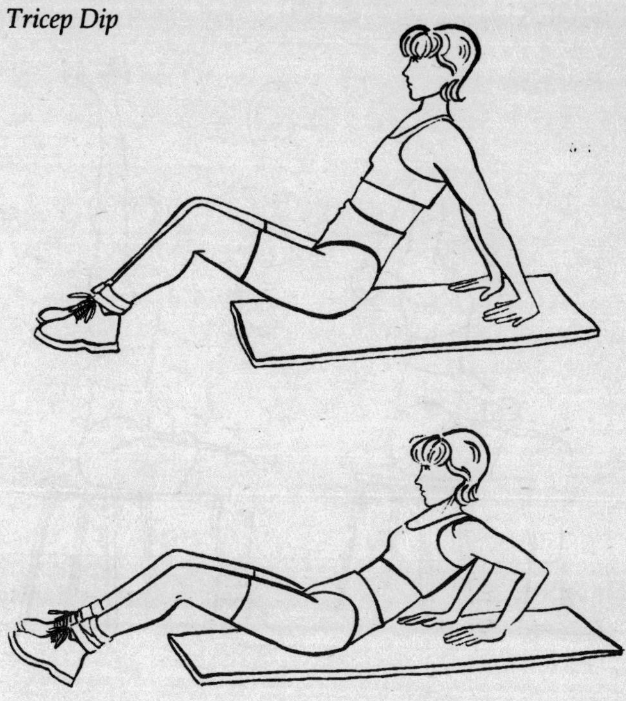

Sit on the floor with your knees bent. Place your hands behind you, making sure that they are as far from the body as you can comfortably reach. The fingers must face forward and the palms of the hands lie flat on the floor. Pull the tummy in to support the back. Make sure the elbows face behind you and lower the body weight back onto the arms as you bend the elbows. Straighten the arms and repeat as many times as you can until you really feel the muscles have worked.

Tricep Extension

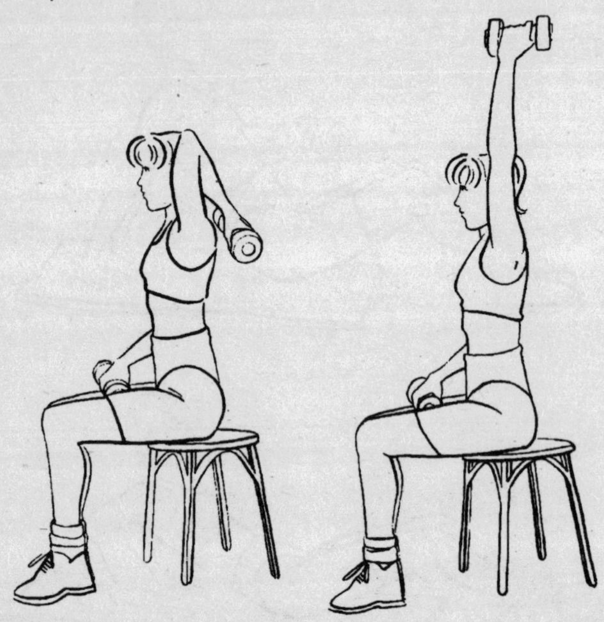

Sit upright either on the floor or in a chair. Touch your left shoulder with your left arm, so that the elbow faces upwards. Hold a tin of beans or a small bottle of water to make it more challenging. Straighten the arm and bend again.

Repeat as many times as you can until you really feel the muscles have worked.

Stretch

Triceps

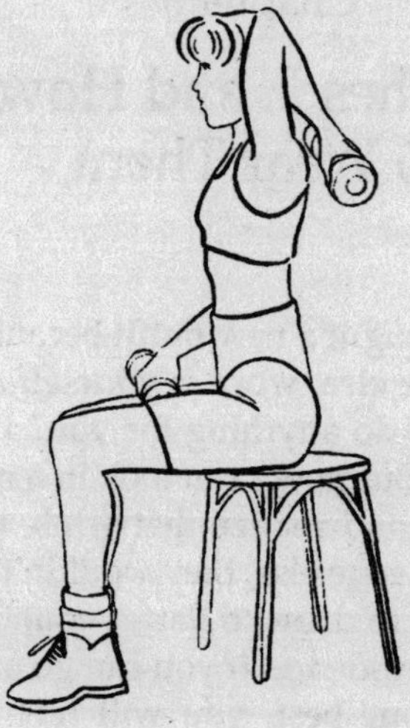

Reach up with the left hand and bend the elbow so that your left hand is touching your left shoulder. Using the right hand, gently ease the arm back. Hold for 10 seconds. Change arms.

Part 4: Dress to Impress

Chapter 8

Clothes ... and How to Wear Them

Have you ever bought a new outfit because it looked great on someone else, worn it yourself and known that it just didn't do anything for you? I have done this many times! But now I can look in a magazine or a shop at outfits and realize that while they would look great on someone else, they wouldn't suit me.

Learning how to dress to flatter your shape gives you enormous confidence. If you can go out knowing that you look your best, you will feel happy and relaxed.

I have a good friend, Carol, who is 6 foot 2 inches (1.88 m) tall. She is very elegant and always looks wonderful. I found myself trying to imitate her style, because I wanted to look wonderful as well, but it seemed no matter what I tried I could never carry off the styles she wore so well. Hardly surprising when you think that I am 5 foot 3 inches (1.55 m) tall with completely different proportions! Once I learned to make the best of my individual statistics, I looked and felt much better.

It is sad but true that most people would rather look like someone else. However, we can *all* make the best of the shape we have got by choosing clothes that flatter our figure and avoiding styles that highlight or emphasize our weakest points.

We are, of course, all individual and although we love to categorize ourselves, we are all actually a combination of many different features. So the guidelines in this section are just that – guidelines. Experiment and see what works best for you. Set aside a couple of hours when you won't be disturbed, get a full length mirror and go through your wardrobe trying on different combinations that you haven't worn together before. There's no need to rush out and spend a fortune – you probably already have a lot of the garments or accessories in the wardrobe that you can use. You may find that you already do some of the things suggested, but if not, try them and see what a difference it makes – you will be pleasantly surprised! Clothes should be fun. Of course they need to be functional and practical, but there's no reason why we can't all dress with style, even if we are just going to the supermarket!

As we now know, most people who are overweight store their excess fat either on their hips, bottom and thighs or in the middle around the tummy. This gives us the traditional apple and pear shapes. Although there are certain aspects of choosing the right styles that are common to both shapes, there are many designs that will flatter one more than the other.

APPLES

Because your overall shape is round, you must be careful not to emphasize the roundness of your tummy with circular lines and seams. The way you dress should ideally emphasize your face. When people see you, you want them to notice your eyes and your smile, not the shape or colour of your jacket.

NECKLINES

Avoid	*Choose*
Large round necklines	Small round narrow lines, *e.g.* turtle or polo neck
Off the shoulder seams	Light shoulder pads
Chunky fabrics	Several lighter layers

COLLARS AND LAPELS

Avoid	*Choose*
Large round shapes	Mid to narrow streamlines

N.B. If you are broad shouldered, choose collars that point down; if you are narrow shouldered, wear collars that point outwards.

WAISTLINE

Avoid	*Choose*
Belts	Longer tops
An obvious break in colour, e.g. bright top and dark skirt with a tight-fitting waist	Slightly higher waisted designs
Dropped-waist dresses	Waistcoats that finish at hip level

HIPS

Avoid	*Choose*
Tight-fitting clothes e.g. leggings	Free flowing designs, slightly streamline, but not too straight
Straight skirts	Medium or longer length skirts

PATTERNS

Avoid	*Choose*
Horizontal stripes	Narrow vertical stripes
	Medium size prints
Large prints (unless you are tall)	Plain colours, especially for tops
Busy designs on top	

GENERAL TIPS

Choose soft, freely flowing fabrics.
Avoid tight-fitting clothes of any style.
Jackets and waistcoats can be used to lower the line of the waist.
Scarves can be loosely draped to hang down, as long as they are not too full. Narrow scarves can be tied around the neck in a ruff-like style if you are wearing a small round-necked jacket.
Several layers of light fabric are better than one thick layer.

PEARS

Because your overall body line is bottom heavy, you must be careful not to choose designs that emphasize this. Instead you need to emphasize your top half more. As with the apple shapes, you should aim to choose clothes that highlight your face rather than your body type.

NECKLINES

Avoid	*Choose*
Narrow V or round necks, unless used with a scarf or wrap	Wider V necks Off the shoulder seams Square necks (unless broad shouldered)

COLLARS AND LAPELS

Avoid	*Choose*
Narrow streamlines	Slightly wider or squarer lines

N.B. if you are broad shouldered, choose collars that point down; if you are narrow shouldered, try collars that point outwards.

WAISTLINE

Avoid	*Choose*
Belts	Looser fitting tops
Dropped waists (hip length)	Mid length tops, i.e just above hip height
Cropped tops	

HIPS

Avoid	*Choose*
Tight-fitting clothes e.g. leggings (unless with a longer top)	Loose-fitting styles
A-line skirts	Fuller, straighter skirts, e.g. pleated
Large pockets on the hips or bottom	Medium to long skirts
Short skirts	

PATTERNS

Avoid	*Choose*
Horizontal stripes on the bottom	Dark or plain bottoms
Large prints on the bottom	Medium-sized patterns for tops

GENERAL TIPS

Avoid heavy fabrics, particularly on the bottom. Fabric must flow freely from the waistline.

Avoid tight-fitting clothes of any style.
Jackets can be used to take the attention away from the hip.
Scarves and accessories can be used to highlight the top half of the body. Brooches, etc., should be worn high on collars and lapels.
Aim to emphasize the top half of your body, and keep the lower half in plain and darker colours.

Whatever your shape, or whichever style works best for you, wear it with confidence. Choosing clothes is a very personal decision, and although I have given you some basic guidelines, if you feel something looks good on you, wear it!

Colours also have a big impact on our image. I have dark hair and a clear, pinkish skin, which means I can wear colours that are quite dramatic, such as red or purple. If I wear pastel shades, however, I look very pale and drawn. Why not treat yourself to a colour analysis when you achieve the dress size you want to be? That will complete the new look – the new you!

Part 5: Enjoy your Meal

Chapter 9

The Practicalities of Healthy Shopping

With the best intentions in the world, you can only eat the foods you buy. In other words, your weight loss programme has to begin in the supermarket. You need to learn how to fill your cupboards with lots of delicious foods that can be quick and easy to prepare, so that when temptation strikes, you have a healthy alternative to the biscuit tin or the local fish and chip shop!

USING YOUR FREEZER

Of course we all know that fresh organic vegetables are probably the most nutritious foods that you can buy. However this does not help much if all you have left in the cupboard is a dried cabbage. Not very appetizing! So make sure you have a good supply of frozen vegetables. I find spinach in particular freezes well and retains its taste and tinned spinach is great for curries. Other vegetables that freeze well include sweetcorn, petit pois and broccoli. It is also useful to keep some bags of frozen mixed vegetables, which can be used for stews and casseroles, particularly if they contain root vegetables such as swede, parsnips and carrots.

Fruit doesn't always freeze that well; strawberries

in particular go very mushy when defrosted. However, many of the summer fruits such as blackcurrants will keep well. Again, these can be brought in bags containing a selection of different summer fruits, which are ideal for fruit salads, or served on their own with some low-fat yoghurt or fromage frais for a quick and easy dessert.

Meat, of course, freezes well. I find it much easier to cut the fat off meat when it is still very cold. Fish also freezes well. If you have poached some fish, freeze the stock, as it can be used as stock in other fish recipes or in a fish soup.

I recommend that you try to reduce the amount of meat you eat by at least a third, progressing to a half over a period of time. The recipes in this book will show you how to cook with less meat and more vegetables, and after a short time, you will be able to adapt the meals you already cook in the same way. You will feel much healthier, lose weight and spend less on shopping – what more could you want?

Most of us keep bread in the freezer and I have found pitta bread to be extremely useful. It can be defrosted in a couple of minutes in the microwave or under a low heat on the grill and can be filled with anything from salad to chicken curry! Personally I prefer pitta bread to any other, as I have found it doesn't cause the bloating that other breads can.

USING YOUR FRIDGE

I can't stress enough the importance of including a selection of raw vegetables in your diet and I have found the best way to do this is to keep a large bowl of green salad in the fridge *(see pages 175 –8 for recipe)*.

I make sure I have a large handful of this every day, either in pitta bread mixed with tuna or salmon, or as an accompaniment to whatever my main meal is. If you want something really quick and easy and don't mind paying a little more, try buying a large bag of ready made salad from the supermarket and a bag of spinach leaves and mixing them together. Choose salad packs that contain watercress and other leaves, not just lettuce. From a nutritional point of view, the lettuce will provide you with the least amount of nutrients, so include as many other vegetables as possible.

Seeds should also be stored in the fridge, preferably in a dark container or jar. Sesame seeds are great for sprinkling over salad (and very rich in calcium) or for adding to a stir fry. Or you could sprinkle a few on your cereal or in a yoghurt. Just a teaspoon per day will be all you need.

FILL UP YOUR CUPBOARDS

Your cupboards should contain:

Rice. Wholegrain or wild rice is especially good.
Pasta, preferably from durum wheat. If you think you may have IBS symptoms you should avoid wheat pasta. Try corn pasta as an alternative or ask in your local health food shop. *(See page 52 for more details on IBS.)*
A selection of stock cubes and purées. I find vegetable purée good for stews and casseroles as it isn't too strong.
A little wine for adding to recipes for extra flavour.
A good selection of herbs and spices. If you are going

to use less meat, you really want to bring out the taste of the vegetables and other ingredients in your recipes. Dried herbs are best kept in the dark, in sealed containers. If they are stale, they will add nothing to the flavour of the food.

...AND VEGETABLE RACK

Your vegetable rack should be constantly full. Remember that potatoes start to sprout if stored in direct sunlight, so keep them in a brown bag if possible. Avoid green potatoes. Onions are also best stored in the dark. Vegetables should be stored for a relatively short period of time, so rather than buying a week's supply at one time, try to buy them every few days.

...AND FRUIT BOWL

Your fruit bowl should also remain well stocked. I recommend up to five pieces of fruit per day, certainly two as a minimum. You can either have fruit as part of a meal – for example, I like to add chopped fruit to my cereal or to have it with a bio-yoghurt – or you can have it on its own as a snack. Tinned fruit can also be used, but avoid varieties in syrup or with added sugar. Buy fruit in natural juice.

COOKING UTENSILS

You will also need a wok or a heavy based pan for cooking. Non-stick varieties are great because you have to add little or no oil. Stir fries can be cooked in just a little water with a dessertspoonful of olive oil. Enamel pans that you can start to cook the food in and then transfer to the oven are also very useful and save on the washing up!

Once you get used to buying more vegetables and fruit, using more rice and flavouring your food with herbs and spices instead of the fat from the meat, you will have transformed your diet into one that will not only help you to lose weight and keep it off, but will also be nutritious and delicious! You won't feel as though you are 'on a diet' at all. The whole family can enjoy the same foods and healthy eating becomes a way of life, not just something you do for a few weeks until you achieve your goal.

Now you've filled your cupboards, let's turn to the recipes themselves.

Chapter 10

The TLC 28-Day Diet

You will find all these recipes delicious and nutritious. Not only that, but they will also help you tone up, lose weight and change shape at the same time!

I suggest you read through the recipes and make a shopping list of the ingredients you will need for the first few days or week. (Remember to buy vegetables every few days if possible.) If some of the recipes contain flavours you don't like, simply leave them out or use an alternative. For example, if you don't like garlic, just use black pepper and some alternative flavourings such as mixed herbs. I have found that the best recipes for me are those that I have adapted to suit my family's individual tastes.

Ideally, you should follow the recipes in the order that they appear here. However if this is not practical, use this chapter as a recipe book and select whatever meal you want.

THE TLC DIET

Hopefully by now you have kept a food log for a few days and can tell roughly how much fat, protein and, most importantly, carbohydrate you are eating on a daily basis. You may feel that you now know enough to adapt your own recipes in order to achieve the right balance. If not, then the following

28 days' worth of suggestions will be enough for you to get a good idea of what you need to achieve. Remember, this is *not* a diet as such, but a way of cooking that will provide your body with lots of nutrients – and will help you lose weight and keep it off.

BREAKFAST

I have not listed 28 different breakfasts! But I do make the following recommendations.

Breakfast is crucial; it helps your metabolism to get going for the day. A sluggish metabolism makes it much harder to lose weight, so *don't* skip breakfast.

If you have not been having breakfast, then you may find that as soon as you do start to have it, you feel hungry for the rest of the morning. This is a normal reaction and it won't last long. Try to resist reaching into the biscuit barrel if you do feel a genuine hunger pang – have a piece of fruit instead. Once your body is used to being fed in the mornings, it will be satisfied until lunch time.

Breakfast suggestions:

Cereals

Try a large bowl of the cereal of your choice, except those containing large quantities of nuts or large quantities of sugar. Try to go for porridge oats if you can, or something similar. There are several 'healthy' breakfast cereals now on the market, but do read the label before you buy. Always choose those with the lowest fat *and* the lowest sugar, irrespective of what it says on the front of the box. Don't always be influenced by cereals, or any other products, that are advertised by athletes or so-called 'healthy' people. It does not guarantee a good quality product.

Home-Made Muesli

This is generally much healthier and certainly much cheaper than shop brought varieties. Use the following ingredients to make up as much or as little as you require. You can make up an individual bowlful each morning or make up a large quantity and keep it in an airtight container, just adding the fresh banana or some other fruit of your choice to it each day. You can experiment with the amount of each ingredient until you find the combination you like the most. If you don't like one of the ingredients, simply leave it out.

Ingredients for home-made muesli:

wheat flakes
oat flakes
barley
almonds (allow a teaspoonful per bowl)
chopped dates
raisins
sunflower seeds (allow a teaspoonful per bowl)
sliced banana or other fruit of your choice.

Serve with skimmed or semi-skimmed milk, or a low-fat fromage frais or yoghurt.

Fruit

Fresh Fruit Salad

This can be made and kept for two or three days in the fridge in an airtight container. You can select any fruit you like, but try to choose a variety of colours and textures, for example:

melon
strawberries
apples
pineapple
grapes
kiwi fruit
peaches
pears

Serve with skimmed or semi-skimmed milk, or a low-fat fromage frais or yoghurt. Banana is also nice in fruit salad, but needs to be added fresh each day. If you use tinned fruit, make sure you buy the varieties in natural juice and not in syrup. Also remember that using a dark tin of fruit, such as raspberries or cherries, will discolour all the other fruit.

Alternatively, if you are in a rush, you could just have two or three pieces of fruit. Again, try not to have three pieces of the same, e.g. three apples.

Bread

Providing you are not having any signs of bloating, then bread is fine for breakfast. Try to select wholemeal or wholegrain varieties and have two thick slices. It is not the bread that is fattening, but what you put on it, so choose carefully. I recommend a little organic honey, jam or marmite. Toppings to avoid are peanut butter (which is 75 per cent fat), cheese and chocolate spreads. A *scrape* of butter is OK, but not lashings.

The fat content of bread:

croissants: 50 per cent fat
poppadoms, fried: 41 per cent fat
chappati: 35 per cent fat
naan: 34 per cent fat
wholemeal: 10 per cent fat
brown: 8 per cent fat
rye: 7 per cent fat
white: 7 per cent fat
poppadoms, raw (grilled): 6 per cent fat
chappati without fat: 5 per cent fat
pitta, white: 4 per cent fat
bagel: 4 per cent fat (may vary for different varieties, e.g. sesame)

As you can see, bagels make an excellent choice, either for breakfast or as a snack.

LUNCH

For lunch, you should choose one of the following:

Sandwich
Using bread (rye bread if wheat is a problem), a filled bagel or a crisp bread. If you need to add butter, use just a scrape. Recommended fillings:

hummus *(for home-made hummus, see recipe p.170)* and cucumber, or watercress
tuna fish (in spring water or brine) with watercress or cucumber
salmon (not in oil) with watercress or cucumber
cottage cheese and finely chopped apple
salad *(see salad recipes, pp.175–8)*
chicken salad (lean cuts only)

banana
tomato

Hummus Recipe
400 g/14 oz chick peas, blended (with a fork or in a blender) for a smooth texture
150–200 g/5–7 oz low-fat fromage frais or plain yoghurt
pinch of black pepper and lemon juice to taste
1 clove garlic, finely chopped

Mix all the ingredients together in a bowl and place in the fridge to cool.

Toast

A real favourite for lunch, because it is quick and easy. Use rye or corn bread if wheat is a problem. If you need to use butter, just have a scrape. Try one of the following toppings:

any of the above sandwich fillings
tinned tomatoes with a pinch of basil
baked beans (low sugar)

Soup

Home-made soups are very simple to make, providing you have a blender or liquidizer. You can use almost any vegetables and vary the soups according to season. In summer you can make a thinner soup by using more water. In winter you may wish to use less water and make a thicker, broth type of soup. You can also vary the spices or herbs you use. I like to add a little chilli powder to spice some of the soups up a little. However if you prefer a less spicy taste, leave it out.

Green Soup
(Leek, Potato and Broccoli)
Suitable for spring clean

4 medium potatoes, finely chopped
½ a large or 1 small leek
3 cups broccoli
1–2 cloves garlic
salt and pepper
water
sage

1 Place the potatoes and leek into boiling water, cover and simmer for 15 minutes.
2 Chop and add the broccoli and the garlic and sage and simmer for a further 10–15 minutes.
3 Blend the mixture and serve.
4 Add extra water to get the desired thickness, reheat thoroughly and serve.
Can be frozen.

Mixed Vegetable Soup
Suitable for spring clean

2 large carrots, finely chopped
1 large parsnip
1 turnip
1 onion, finely chopped
1 cup cabbage, finely chopped

salt and pepper
2 tsp fresh coriander, chopped

1. Place all the vegetables into a large pan of boiling water, cover and simmer for 20–30 minutes or until soft, adding the coriander, salt and pepper after 15 minutes.
2. Blend the mixture.
3. Add extra water to get the desired thickness, reheat thoroughly and serve.
   Can be frozen.

Carrot, Courgette and Sweetcorn Soup

Suitable for spring clean

2 large carrots
2 courgettes
1 cup sweetcorn
1 onion, finely chopped
salt and pepper
½–1 tsp oregano

1. Place the carrots into a large pan of boiling water, cover and simmer for 10 minutes.
2. Add the courgettes and onions and simmer for a further 10 minutes.
3. Add the sweetcorn, salt and pepper and oregano and simmer for a further 5 minutes.
4. Blend.
5. Add extra water to get the desired thickness, heat thoroughly and serve.
   Can be frozen.

Vegetable and Lentil Soup

Suitable for spring clean

2 large carrots
1 onion, finely chopped
1 cup red lentils, cooked as per packet instructions
2 sticks celery, finely chopped
½ tsp cumin
½ tsp coriander
salt and pepper

1. Add the carrots to a large pan of boiling water, cover and simmer for 10 minutes.
2. Add the onion and the celery, simmer for a further 5 minutes.
3. Add the lentils, salt and pepper and herbs, and simmer very gently for 5 minutes.
4. Blend.
5. Add extra water to get the desired thickness and serve.
   Can be frozen.

Spicy Soup

2 large carrots
1 parsnip
225 g/8 oz tomatoes, finely chopped (can use tinned for speed)
1 225 g/8 oz tin mixed beans in spicy sauce
1 large stick celery
1 onion, finely chopped
2 cloves garlic

½ small green chilli or ½ tsp chilli powder
parsley to garnish

1 Place the carrots and parsnips into a large pan of boiling water, cover and simmer for 10 minutes.
2 Add the onion and the cloves of garlic and simmer for a further 10 minutes.
3 Blend the mixture.
4 Return to the pan and add the tomatoes, beans and chilli. Simmer gently for about 5 minutes.
5 Add extra water to get the desired thickness and serve with parsley on top.
Can be frozen.

Jacket Potato

Have a large potato, with one of the following fillings:

tuna fish (in brine or spring water) mixed with a pinch of coriander (optional)
salmon mixed with a pinch of coriander or dill (optional)
baked beans (low sugar if possible)
hot tinned tomatoes with a pinch of mixed herbs
hot tinned tomatoes mixed with sliced mushrooms or tuna fish (in brine or spring water)
tuna (in brine or spring water) and sweetcorn
hummus with chopped cucumber and or watercress
cottage cheese with chopped apple or pineapple
mixed bean salad, drained
stir fry mixed vegetables: slice ½ carrot, ½ cup mangetout and ½ stick celery and gently fry in ½ tsp olive oil and 1 tbsp water; add soy sauce to taste

sweetcorn and pineapple
one of the salad recipes *(see below)*

LIVELY, DELICIOUS SALAD RECIPES

People think of salad as being boring – not so! Salad can be not only very nutritious, but also delicious. If you are used to lettuce, onion, cucumber and tomato salads, then try the following recipes and you will never feel the same about salad again!

Use the ingredients suggested in varying amounts according to taste. Salad can be kept in the fridge in an airtight container for three days. It can be served with tuna fish, salmon or a little lean meat, e.g. chicken or turkey, or in a jacket potato *(see above)*.

Dressings

A dressing is shown with each salad. However, these are only guidelines and you can chop and change which dressing goes with which salad according to your taste. Another natural dressing is shown in the spring clean section on page 100. This may also be used with any of the salads.

Green Salad

crisp lettuce
grapefruit segments
sliced courgettes
mangetout
green beans

Suggested dressing
Mix together the following ingredients: low-fat fromage frais, salt and pepper, coarse wholegrain mustard and a drop of skimmed milk if necessary.

Carrot and Orange Salad

spinach leaves
carrot, finely grated
green pepper, finely sliced
celery, finely chopped
orange segments (can be replaced with melon or pineapple if preferred)
chopped parsley

Suggested Dressing
Mix together the following ingredients: the juice of 1 orange (or lemon for a more bitter taste) mixed with low-fat natural yoghurt, parsley, a little salt and black pepper.

Chinese Salad

pineapple segments
lettuce
beansprouts
Chinese leaf
spring onion
chicory
cucumber, cut into strips

Suggested Dressing
Mix together the following ingredients: wine vinegar, ½ tsp olive oil, ½ tsp sesame oil, a sprinkling of sesame seeds.

Red Salad

red cabbage
radichio
onion (sliced)
red apple (keep the peel on)
celery

Suggested Dressing
Mix the following ingredients together: low-fat yoghurt or fromage frais, a little cider vinegar, finely chopped garlic, salt and pepper.

Summer Salad

lettuce
sliced cucumber
fresh strawberries
mangetout

Suggested Dressing
Mix the following ingredients together: low-fat yoghurt or fromage frais, a little vinegar, chopped fresh mint and black pepper.

Vegetable Salad

spinach leaves
chopped broccoli
chopped cauliflower
mangetout
cherry tomatoes
sliced green peppers

Suggested Dressing
Mix together the following ingredients: low-fat yoghurt or fromage frais, chopped mint.

DAY 1

Chicken or Vegetable Nasi Goreng

Serves 4

300 g/10 oz rice
1 tsp sesame oil
a large dash of teriyaki sauce
250 g/9 oz root vegetables of your choice, chopped into tiny chunks
1 large carrot, sliced
1 green or red pepper, sliced
2 tsp 5 spice powder
pinch coriander
pinch cayenne pepper
1 dstsp of finely chopped ginger
2 cloves garlic
4 tbsp soy sauce
200 g/7 oz beansprouts

Meat Option: Replace 100 g/3 oz of the vegetables with 200 g/7 oz of sliced chicken.

1 Put the rice on to cook.
2 Gently heat the oil in a large pan and a cup of water. Add the garlic and ginger and fry for 2 minutes.
3 Add the root vegetables and teriyaki sauce and stir fry for 5 minutes. Cover and simmer over a low heat for a further 10 minutes or until vegetables are soft. (If you cut them very small it will take less time.) Drain off excess water.
4 Add the carrot and pepper and stir fry for a further 2–3 minutes.
5 Add the 5 spice powder, soy sauce, beansprouts, coriander and pepper and continue to stir fry for a further 3–4 minutes.

Add the chicken after stage 2. You can also marinate the chicken in a little teriyaki sauce for a stronger flavour before you add the water. Stir fry for 3–4 minutes.
Serve with green salad.

DAY 2

American Meat/Vegetable Loaf

200 g/7 oz lean minced beef (can be substituted with turkey if preferred)
40 g/1 oz oats
2 large carrots, grated

1 large parsnip, grated
1 large courgette, grated
1 finely chopped onion
dstsp tomato purée
dash Worcester sauce
pinch mace or nutmeg
3 tbsp skimmed milk or vegetable stock (less if using all vegetables)
fresh or dried herbs to taste
1 egg, beaten
1 kg/2 lb loaf tin, very lightly greased
If you do not want to use meat, replace with 200 g/ 7 oz grated root vegetables of your choice.

Preheat oven to 180°C/350°F/gas mark 4.

1. Mix all the ingredients together; knead and bind together with the egg.
2. Cook for about 1½ hours or until cooked.

Can be eaten hot or cold. This dish also freezes very well.
Serve with new potatoes and vegetables of your choice or with a green salad and rice if eaten cold.

DAY 3

Shepherd's Pie

Serves 4

400 g/14 oz vegetables of your choice, e.g. carrots, parsnips, swede, celery or courgettes, chopped

1 large tin mixed beans (in spicy sauce if preferred)
1 large tin tomatoes
1 large onion
2 cloves garlic
125 g/4 oz mushrooms
1 tbsp vegetable purée
salt and pepper
pinch marjoram
pinch basil
600 g/1½ lb mixture of potatoes and parsnips
2 tbsp low-fat fromage frais
1 dstsp olive oil and the same of water
For meat, replace 200 g/7 oz vegetables with 200 g/7 oz lean mince (beef or turkey).

Preheat oven to 200°C/400°F/gas mark 6.

1. Peel and chop the potatoes and the parsnips and put on to boil.
2. Gently heat the oil and water, and fry the onion and garlic.
3. Add the tin of tomatoes and the vegetables, including mushrooms, and the seasoning.
4. Cook gently for 10 minutes. Add a little vegetable stock if the mixture seems too dry.
5. Add the tin of beans, stir well and cook for a further 5 minutes.
6. Place the mixture into an ovenproof dish.
7. Mash the potatoes and parsnips together, and add the fromage frais. Spread this mixture over the top of the filling and place in the oven for 30 minutes. Increase the oven temperature to 230°C/450°F/gas mark 8 for a further 10 minutes to brown the potato topping.

If using meat, add the mince after stage 2 and continue as given.

Serve with a dark green vegetable or other vegetable of your choice.

DAY 4

Turkey or Vegetable Stir Fry

Serves 4

2 tsp sesame oil with water
2½ cm/1 inch piece of root ginger, peeled and grated
3 cloves garlic, chopped (can reduce to 1 clove if preferred)
1 fresh chilli, finely chopped
1 onion, chopped
600 g/1½ lb mixed vegetables of your choice, washed and chopped
3 tbsp soy sauce
1 packet thread egg noodles/rice noodles
1 tbsp black bean sauce
1 tbsp oyster sauce
If you are using meat, 250 g/9 oz minced turkey in place of 250 g/9 oz vegetables.

1. Gently heat the oil and water in a large pan, and stir fry the garlic, ginger, chilli and onion.
2. Add the vegetables and continue to stir fry.
3. Add the soy sauce, black bean sauce and oyster sauce, and continue to cook over a gentle heat.

4 Cook the noodles according to the instructions on the packet, drain and add to the stir fry. Toss well and serve.
If using turkey, add at stage 1 and continue as given.

Serve with salad.

DAY 5

Grilled Plaice with Roasted Vegetables

Serves 4

4 plaice fillets
1 red pepper, sliced
8–10 whole baby sweetcorn
100 g/3 oz mangetout
2 large carrots, cut into strips
1 425 g/15 oz tin of tomatoes
pinch tarragon
salt and pepper
a sprinkling of soy sauce

Preheat oven to 190°C/375°F/gas mark 5.

1. Place all the vegetables in a ceramic dish with a lid and pour over the tin of tomatoes.
2. Add the tarragon, soy sauce and seasoning, and stir well, so that all the vegetables are covered with tomato.
3. Place the fish on top of the vegetables, put the lid on the dish and place in the oven.

4 Bake for about 30 minutes or until fish is cooked.

Serve with the vegetables and new potatoes or a large jacket potato.

DAY 6

Vegetable/Meat Curry Special

Serves 4

600 g/1½ pounds of mixed vegetables of your choice, e.g. carrots, beans, potatoes, cauliflower
25–50 g/1–2 oz red lentils (cook as per packet instructions)
1 onion
1 glove garlic
25 g/1 oz root ginger
1 dstsp olive oil and the same of water
2 tbsp curry powder or paste
300 ml/½] pint vegetable stock (use vegetable water if possible, if not use a cube)
125 g/4 oz low-fat natural yoghurt
2 dstsps lemon juice
Meat Option: Replace 200 g/7 oz of vegetables with 200 g/7 oz chicken.

Boil water in a large pan and cook brown rice for approx. 45 minutes. Whilst this is cooking, prepare and cook the curry:

1 Gently heat the oil and water and sauté the

onion, garlic and ginger until the onion is transparent. Add the curry powder or paste.

2 Slowly pour in the vegetable stock and bring to the boil. Add the vegetables and cook gently for about 20–30 minutes. (If you have used root vegetables it will take 30–40 minutes, if not 20–30.)
3 Blend the lemon juice with a little of the sauce from the pot and stir in slowly.
4 A few minutes before serving, stir in the yoghurt. Do not boil.

If using chicken, gently stir fry over a low heat for 4–5 mins and add after stage 1.
Serve with the rice and a green salad, and low-fat yoghurt with chopped cucumber.

DAY 7

Chicken or Bean Casserole

Serves 4

1 large aubergine, chopped
salt and pepper
2 red peppers, chopped
1 dstsp olive oil and the same of water
1 large onion, chopped
2 cloves garlic
3–4 medium courgettes, sliced
425 g/15 oz tin tomatoes
425 g/15 oz tin beans (flagolet or mixed), drained
300 g/10 oz cauliflower

200 g/7 oz button mushrooms
1 dstsp tomato purée
1 tsp crushed coriander seeds
Meat Option: Replace cauliflower with 200 g/7 oz chicken.

1. Place the chopped aubergine into a colander and sprinkle with salt. Leave for 30 minutes to take away the bitterness.
2. Gently heat the oil and water and sauté the onion for 3–4 minutes.
3. Rinse the aubergine and pat dry. Add to the onions, with the garlic and peppers. Cook over a gentle heat for 10 minutes.
4. Add the courgettes, cauliflower, mushrooms, tomatoes and tomato purée and cook for 15 minutes over a gentle heat.
5. Add the beans and coriander and cook gently for a further 5 minutes. Add pepper to taste.
   If using chicken, add after stage 2.

Serve with a large jacket potato, or other potato of your choice, and a dark green vegetable such as spinach or broccoli.

DAY 8

Fish Cakes

Serves 4

1 175 g/6 oz tin of skinless, boneless tuna or salmon in water or brine

1 onion, finely chopped
2 slices wholemeal (or rye) bread in crumbs
1 egg, beaten
2 tbsp fresh parsley, chopped
flour for dusting
1 tsp olive oil and the same of water
1 lemon rind and juice
1 tsp dill or coriander

1. Drain the fish.
2. Gently heat the oil and water in a pan and sauté the onion for 3–4 minutes until transparent.
3. Place the fish, the onion, lemon juice, herbs and breadcrumbs in a mixing bowl.
4. Add the beaten egg and bind together.
5. Divide into patties and lightly dust with the flour. Return to the pan and fry over a gentle heat for about 3 minutes each side or until lightly browned.

Serve with new potatoes or oven chips *(see page 208)* and a green salad or green vegetable.

DAY 9

Vegetable/Chicken Kebabs with Pilaff

Serves 4

1 dstsp olive oil with 1 dstsp water
1 apple, chopped
1 large onion, chopped
2 large sticks celery, chopped

200 g/7 oz brown rice
600 ml/1 pint vegetable stock (use vegetable water if possible, if not use a cube)
50 g/2 oz seedless raisins
50 g/2 oz dried apricots, chopped
1 cinnamon stick (or ½–1 tsp powder)
1 bay leaf
salt and pepper
kebabs (vegetable)
200 g/7 oz courgettes, cut into chunks
8 small tomatoes
1 large onion, cut into wedges
½ green pepper, cut into large pieces
½ red pepper, cut into pieces
1½–2 tsp olive oil
1 dstsp thyme
Meat Kebabs: Use 2 chicken breasts, cut into cubes, to replace the courgettes.

Pilaff

1. Gently heat the oil and water in a large pan.
2. Add the onion and the celery and gently fry for 4–5 mins
3. Add the rice and cook for 1–2 minutes, stirring all the time.
4. Pour over the vegetable stock, and add the raisins and apricots and chopped apple.
5. Bring to the boil and stir occasionally. Add the bay leaf, cinnamon and salt and pepper.
6. Reduce the heat and cover. Simmer for about 30 minutes or until the rice is soft and the stock absorbed.

Kebabs

1 Whilst the pilaff is cooking, place the courgettes in a pan of boiling water and blanch for 1 minute, then drain.
2 Place the vegetables onto skewers, alternating tomatoes, onions and peppers.
3 Mix together the oil and thyme and brush over the kebabs. Grill for about 10 minutes, turning frequently.
Meat Option: Cut 2 large chicken breasts into cubes to replace courgettes. Prepare in the same way, except grill for slightly longer if necessary.

To serve, arrange the pilaff in a dish and place the kebabs on top. Serve with a green salad.

DAY 10

Meat or Bean Hot Pot

Serves 4

2–3 cups of macaroni or corn pasta
2 large 425 g/15 oz tins red kidney beans or mixed beans in a spicy sauce
1 green pepper
150 g/5 oz mushrooms
2 large tomatoes
100 g/3 oz red lentils (cooked as per instructions on packet)
2 large courgettes
1 large leek
1 medium onion

1 dstsp olive oil, with the same of water
2½ cm/1 inch chilli, or chilli powder (optional)
juice and rind of 1 orange (optional)

N.B. The chilli powder and the orange give the dish a much spicier and fruitier flavour.

Meat Option: Replace 1 tin of beans and 1 courgette with 200 g/7 oz lean beef, cubed, or other meat of your choice.

1 Cook the macaroni or pasta as per packet instructions.
2 Gently heat the oil and water, and fry the onion and pepper for 2 minutes.
3 Add the mushrooms, courgettes, leek and tomatoes and cook for a further 10 minutes.
4 Add the lentils, chilli powder (optional), orange (optional) and tins of beans. Stir well and cook for a further 10 minutes.
5 Drain and rinse the macaroni or pasta, and combine with the hot pot. Stir well over a gentle heat for a further 2 minutes and serve.

DAY 11

Chicken or Vegetable Risotto

Serves 4

3 large carrots
2 large leeks
2 large courgette

125 g/4 oz button mushrooms
100 g/3 oz cucumber
1–2 cloves garlic
2 large onions, chopped
50 g/2 oz almonds
375 g/12 oz brown rice
900 ml/1½ pints vegetable stock
salt and pepper
1 dstsp olive oil with the same of water
Meat Option: Replace 1 carrot, 1 leek and 1 courgette with 200 g/7 oz chicken fillet, chopped.

1. Wash and slice all the vegetables.
2. Gently heat the oil and water, and sauté the onions and garlic.
3. Add the vegetables and the almonds and continue to stir for 5 minutes.
4. Add the stock, seasoning and rice and boil for 5 minutes.
5. Add the cucumber and reduce the heat. Cover and simmer until the rice is cooked and all the stock absorbed. This will take approximately 40 minutes. To reduce cooking time you may wish to use white rice.

If using chicken, add after stage 2 and continue as given. Serve with a salad of your choice.

DAY 12

Chicken or Tuna or Vegetable Pasta

200 g/7 oz chicken, diced, or 1 200 g/7 oz tin of tuna in water or brine, drained (optional)
1 425 g/15 oz tin chopped tomatoes
100 g/3 oz sliced mushrooms
1 red pepper
1 large onion, chopped
1 glove garlic, chopped
1 tbsp vegetable or tomato purée
50 g/2 oz sweetcorn
1 dstsp olive oil with same of water
500 g/1 lb pasta
large pinch of fresh basil, or mixed herbs or Italian seasoning
salt and black pepper

Cook the pasta as per instructions on the packet.

1 Lightly sauté the onion and garlic in the water and oil.
2 Add the chicken (optional) (do not add the tuna at this stage) and cook gently for about 5 minutes.
3 Add the mushrooms, pepper and purée and continue to stir fry for 2–3 minutes.
4 Add the tomatoes, sweetcorn and seasoning.
5 Add the tuna (optional) (if you are using it in place of chicken).
6 Continue to cook, stirring frequently, for about 5 minutes.

7 Drain the pasta and rinse well with boiling water. Place the pasta in a large bowl and add the sauce. Stir well, so that all the pasta is covered with the sauce.

Serve with a green salad or salad of your choice.

DAY 13

Fruity Chicken or Vegetables

Serves 4

425 g/15 oz tin tomatoes
2 tbsp fruit chutney
50 g/2 oz raisins
25 g/1 oz chopped almonds
½–1 tbsp tabasco sauce
1 tbsp apricot jam
600 g/1½ lb of root vegetables, e.g. carrots, whole baby sweetcorn, mangetout or green beans, celery, red or yellow peppers, swede, etc.
1 onion
2 cloves garlic
1 dstsp olive oil and the same of water
Meat Option: Replace half the vegetables with 2 chicken fillets, diced.

1 Peel and chop the vegetables, and put in a large pan. Barely cover with water and bring to the boil. Cover and simmer gently for 10 minutes.
2 Gently heat the oil and water and fry the onion and garlic for 2 minutes.

3 Drain the vegetables, retaining the stock in case you need it later. Add to the onions and garlic and cook for about 10 minutes. Add the tomatoes. Replace some stock if you like.
4 Add the tabasco sauce, jam, chutney, nuts and raisins and continue to stir over a gentle heat for a further 10 minutes or until the vegetables are soft.
If using meat, add after stage 2 and continue as given.

For a less sweet taste, leave out the apricot jam and use 1 tbsp chutney.
Serve with rice and a green salad.

DAY 14

Beef or Vegetable Stew

Serves 4

400 g/14 oz of vegetables of your choice, e.g. turnips, swede
3 medium onions, chopped
300–600 ml/½–1 pint vegetable stock
150 ml/¼ pint red wine
3 cloves garlic, crushed
1 tbsp tomato or vegetable purée
2 tbsp fresh parsley
2 sticks celery, chopped
1 large carrot, chopped
1 dstsp olive oil and the same of water
1 tbsp rosemary

salt and pepper
1 jar approx. 250 g/9 oz sun dried tomatoes
If using beef, replace 200 g/7 oz of vegetables with 200 g/7 oz lean cubed beef.
Preheat the oven to 180°C/350°F/gas mark 4.

1 Gently heat the oil and water, and fry the onions and garlic with the tomato purée.
2 Add the sun dried tomatoes, stock and wine and simmer for 1 minute.
3 Add all the vegetables, the rosemary and seasoning. Cover and simmer for 5 minutes on a low heat.
4 Put the stew into an ovenproof dish. Place in the oven for 1 hour on a low heat or until meat is tender.
If using meat, add after stage 2.
Serve with mashed or jacket potato.

DAY 15

Ratatouille with Grilled Chicken (Optional)

Serves 4

4 red peppers
1 large onion
2 cloves garlic
3 sun dried tomatoes, chopped
1 large aubergine
2 courgettes
6 large ripe tomatoes
2 tbsp chopped parsley

2 tbsp chopped basil
1 cup vegetable or chicken stock
1 dstsp olive oil and the same of water
salt and pepper
2 chicken fillets, chopped into small pieces (optional)

1 Slice the aubergine and sprinkle with salt. Leave for about 10 minutes, then rinse and pat dry with kitchen towel.
2 Prepare the other vegetables by washing and cutting into wedges or slices.
3 Gently heat the oil and water, and cook the onion wedges for about 1 minute.
4 Add the peppers and continue to stir fry gently for about 2 minutes.
5 Pour in the stock, add the garlic and sun dried tomatoes and bring to the boil.
6 Add the aubergine and courgettes and continue to cook for a further 2–3 minutes.
7 Add the tomatoes and seasonings and simmer for about 10 minutes or until vegetables are soft and the sauce is covering all the vegetables.
   Meat Option: Add the chicken after stage 3 and continue as given.

Serve with rice or a jacket potato and salad.

DAY 16

Chicken/Vegetable Stir Fry

Serves 4

3 tbsp teriyaki sauce
pinch 5 spice powder
1 tbsp dark soy sauce
approx. 250 g/9 oz mixed vegetables of your choice, e.g. broccoli, carrots and courgettes, sliced
2 tsp sesame oil
1 tbsp chopped root ginger
1 glove garlic
1 red pepper, sliced
1 bunch spring onions, cut into strips
1 handful beansprouts
1–2 tbsp sherry
Meat Option: Replace 100 g/3 oz of the vegetables with 200 g/7 oz sliced chicken.

1 Gently heat the oil in a large pan. Add the garlic and ginger and stir fry for 2 minutes. Add the sliced vegetables, pour on the teriyaki sauce and the soy sauce and add the 5 spice powder. Continue to stir fry for 3 or 4 minutes.
2 Add the sherry and the beansprouts. Cover and simmer for 2 minutes.

Meat Option: Place the chicken in a bowl and cover with the teriyaki sauce, soy sauce and 5 spice powder. Leave to stand for at least 20 minutes. Add to the pan after the onions, garlic and ginger, and stir fry for 3–4 minutes before continuing with the

directions above.
Serve with rice.

DAY 17

Tuna and/or Sweetcorn Flan

Serves 4

100 g/3 oz ground almonds
100 g/3 oz butter
salt and pepper
35 g/1½ oz brown rice flour
35 g/1½ oz oatbran

Filling
1 175 g/6 oz tin sweetcorn
150 ml/¼ pint skimmed milk or small pot low-fat yoghurt
1 tbsp fresh parsley, chopped
1 175 g/6 oz tin tuna in spring water or brine (optional)
1 egg
1 onion, finely chopped

Preheat oven to 190°C/375°F/gas mark 5.

1. Mix the ground almonds, brown rice flour and oatbran with a little salt and pepper.
2. Mash together with butter to form a soft dough.
3. Lightly grease a pie or flan dish and press the mixture in to form a solid base and walls.
4. Beat the egg and milk or yoghurt together.

5 Place the tuna (optional), onion and sweetcorn evenly in the dish and season.
6 Sprinkle over the chopped parsley and pour over the egg mixture.
7 Bake for approximately 30 minutes, until pale gold.

Serve with new potatoes or a large jacket potato and salad or a vegetable rice.

DAY 18

Pizza Diane

Serves 4

Named after one of my tutors, this is a delicious pizza that uses potato for the base. Ideal for IBS sufferers.

200 g/7 oz boiled potatoes
100 g/3 oz flour (rye flour if preferred)
salt and pepper
12 g/½ oz butter (for greasing)

Topping

1 150 g/5 oz tin tuna in spring water or brine (optional)
150 g/5 oz low-fat cheese, grated
1 red pepper, thinly sliced
1 tbsp olive oil
2 tsp lemon juice
½ tbsp oregano

1 large onion, chopped
1 clove garlic, chopped
50 g/2 oz frozen sweetcorn
2 tbsp tomato purée
salt and pepper

Preheat the oven to 200°C/400°F/gas mark 6.

1 Boil the potatoes until soft and mash them to a pulp with the butter.
2 Sift in the flour and a little salt and pepper, and mix to form a dough. Transfer to a lightly floured surface and knead gently.
3 Roll out and place onto a *very lightly* greased baking sheet.
4 Gently heat the olive oil and fry the onion, pepper and garlic for 5 minutes.
5 Stir in the sweetcorn, tuna (optional), oregano and lemon juice and add salt and pepper.
6 Spread the tomato purée on the pizza base and top with the onion mixture.
7 Place the cheese on top and bake on a high shelf in the oven for 40 minutes.

Serve with a salad of your choice.

DAY 19

Mackerel with Mustard and Yoghurt Sauce

Serves 4

4 small mackerel fillets

1 tbsp Dijon mustard
1 tbsp fresh parsley, chopped
125 g/4 oz plain low-fat fromage frais
salt and black pepper

1. Lightly grill the mackerel for about 10 minutes or until flesh is cooked.
2. Stir the mustard, salt and pepper and parsley into the fromage frais.
3. Place the mackerel onto a plate and pour over the fromage frais sauce.

Serve immediately with new potatoes or a large jacket potato together with a green salad or vegetables of your choice.

DAY 20

Chinese Vegetable/Meat Special

Serves 4

1 dstsp olive oil and the same of water
2 gloves garlic, chopped
2 large onions, chopped
2 sticks celery, chopped
1 red and 1 green pepper, sliced
¼ head of cabbage or Chinese leaf
large pinch ginger powder
salt and black or red pepper to taste
1½ tsp arrowroot powder
1 cup of beansprouts
Meat Option: Add 2 chicken breasts or 200 g/7 oz

pork and half of all vegetables.

1 Gently heat the oil with 1 dstsp water and add the garlic and onions. Sauté for a few minutes until transparent.
2 Add celery, peppers and half the spices, and cook for 4 minutes.
3 Add the cabbage or Chinese leaf and the rest of the spices, saving a little garlic.
4 Sift the arrowroot and blend with a small amount of cold water. Stir this into the vegetables and cook for about 5 minutes or until mixture thickens.
5 Add the remaining garlic and beansprouts and cook for a further 4 minutes on a low heat.

If using chicken, add at stage 1 and stir fry for approximately 4–5 minutes over a gentle heat. Serve with rice.

DAY 21

Pork/Bean and Vegetable Casserole

Serves 4

2 425 g/15 oz tins of kidney beans, mixed beans or other (alternatively use 225 g/8 oz black beans, soaked overnight)
1 dstsp olive oil and same of water
1 medium onion, chopped
1 green pepper, chopped
1 red chilli, finely chopped (optional)
7 oz long grain brown rice
4 large tomatoes

1 clove garlic, chopped
1 red pepper, sliced
I large stick celery
1 tsp coriander
300 ml/½ pint vegetable stock
salt and pepper
Meat Option: Replace 1 tin of beans with 2 chopped pork fillets.

1 Cook the beans in boiling water for 15 minutes (unless using tinned). Reduce heat, simmer for 45 minutes and drain.
2 Gently fry the onion in the oil and water for 3 minutes. Add the garlic, peppers, celery and chilli. Cook for a further 3 minutes. stirring continually.
3 Add the tomatoes, seasoning and coriander, and cook for 1 minute.
4 Add the rice, vegetable stock and beans, and bring to the boil. Cover and simmer for 45 minutes, until the rice is cooked and the stock has been absorbed.
If using pork, add at stage 2 and continue as given.

Serve with mashed potatoes and parsnips, or a large jacket potato and vegetable of your choice.

DAY 22

Pork Steak with Apples and Onions

Serves 4

4 small boneless pork steaks, trimmed of fat
5 tbsp flour
2 egg whites, lightly whisked
8 tbsp of wholemeal breadcrumbs
2 tbsp of low-fat cheese, grated
1 onion
1 or 2 cloves garlic, finely chopped
4 Granny Smith apples, peeled, cored and sliced
150 ml/¼ pint medium dry cider
salt and pepper

1. Flatten the pork steaks, using a steak hammer or a rolling pin.
2. Have ready the egg white, in a shallow dish, and combine the breadcrumbs with the cheese.
3. Firmly press the steak into the flour, salt and pepper, and coat both sides. Dip each steak in the egg white, covering all areas.
4. For the filling, put the cider and the onion in a saucepan. Add the garlic and cover. Boil until the liquid is almost gone. Add the apples and continue to cook, stirring regularly, until the apples are soft.
5. Grill one side of the steaks on a rack, on high heat. Try to have the meat as close to the top of the grill as possible. Remove from the heat and place a generous helping of the apple mixture on top of the steak. Return to the grill for a further 3 minutes or until the mixture has browned.

Serve with new potatoes and 2 vegetables of your choice.

Vegetarian Option

Stuffed Peppers

Serves 4

4 red or green peppers
1 small onion, finely chopped
3 tbsp cider
4 apples, chopped
mixed dried herbs and seasoning to taste
8 slices of wholemeal bread, in breadcrumbs

1. Cut tops off peppers.
2. Clean the peppers of seeds.
3. Soak the breadcrumbs in the cider.
4. Add herbs and seasoning.
5. Stuff the peppers with the breadcrumb mixture and replace the tops.
6. Bake for 25 mins at 200°C/400°F/gas mark 6.

DAY 23

Lasagne (Meat or Vegetable)

Serves 4

600 g/1½ lb mixed vegetables of your choice, washed and chopped
1 425 g/15 oz tin of tomatoes
1 medium onion, chopped

2 cloves garlic
150–300 ml/¼–½ pint vegetable stock
1 tsp basil
1 tsp oregano
1 bay leaf
3 tbsp red wine
8 sheets lasagne
50 g/2 oz low-fat cheese, grated
50 g/2 oz cornflour
12 g/½ oz butter
150–300/¼–½ pint skimmed milk
100 g/3 oz cottage cheese
salt and pepper
1 dstsp olive oil and the same of water
Meat Option: Replace 200 g/7 oz of vegetables with 200 g/7 oz lean mince.

Preheat the oven to 190°C/375°F/gas mark 5.

1 Gently heat the oil and water, and fry the garlic and onion for 2 minutes.
2 Place the vegetables in a ceramic roasting dish, and add the garlic and onions. Pour over the tinned tomatoes and about half of the stock, including the red wine, and cover. Bake in the oven for about 30 minutes. (N.B. For a quicker version, simply stir fry the vegetables for 10 minutes, adding a little stock to keep the mixture smooth, although roasting the vegetables does give a really nice flavour to the dish.)
3 For the white sauce, place 4 tbsp of the milk into a bowl and add the cornflour. Stir to make a paste.
4 Put the remaining milk and butter into a pan and

heat gently, then add the grated cheese. Do not allow to boil.

5 Remove from the heat and pour the hot mixture onto the cold milk and cornflour. Stir until the sauce is smooth and thickens.
6 Remove the vegetables from the oven and add the seasoning, together with a little more stock if necessary.
7 Transfer the vegetable mixture into a separate bowl. Place a layer of vegetables back into the dish, cover with a layer of lasagne and then a layer of white sauce. Repeat this two or three times, according to the size and depth of your dish.
8 Return to the oven and cook for about 30 minutes. Remove from the oven and cover the top with a thin layer of cottage cheese. Return and cook for a further 5 minutes.

If you are using mince, stir fry it whilst the vegetables are roasting and then mix it with the vegetables when they come out of the oven. Continue as described.

Serve with a green salad or salad of your choice.

DAY 24

Turkey Burgers or Vegi-Burgers

Serves 4

1 dstsp olive oil and the same of water
2 onions

1 green or red peppers, finely chopped
150 g/5 oz tofu
1 tsp mixed herbs
salt and pepper
100 g/3 oz ground almonds or mixed nuts containing almonds
100 g/3 oz wholemeal breadcrumbs
1 egg, beaten
2 tbsp hot vegetable stock
2 tsp tomato purée
Meat Option: Use approx. 200 g/7 oz turkey mince.

1. Gently heat the oil and water in a pan. Sauté the onions for 4 minutes.
2. Add the peppers and cook gently for a further 2–3 minutes.
3. Break the tofu into tiny pieces and sprinkle in. Cook for a further 3 minutes.
4. Mix the herbs with the tomato purée and add to the mixture. Simmer for a further 3–4 minutes on a very low heat.
5. Remove from the heat and add the breadcrumbs, beaten egg and the hot stock and almonds. Bind together and divide into round patties. Place on a baking tray and cook in the oven for about 20 minutes on a moderate heat, 190°C/375°F/gas mark 5.
   If using meat, add after stage 1.

Serve in a wholemeal bun, with green salad and oven chips.

Oven Chips

1. Using a pastry brush, very lightly oil the base of a

roasting tin and place in the oven at approx. 220°C/425°F/gas mark 7.

2 Scrub several large new potatoes and slice into chips.
3 Boil for 5 minutes. Drain and sprinkle with stir fry seasoning (and garlic if you like).
4 Add to the roasting tin and bake the potato chips until brown.

DAY 25

Meat or Vegetable Cobbler

Serves 4

3 large carrots
1 tbsp cornflour
2 tbsp fresh parsley
½ small cauliflower
3 leeks (cook in water and save as stock)
150 ml/¼ pint vegetable stock (from leeks)
50 g/2 oz sweetcorn
Meat Option: Add two chicken fillets, chopped into cubes, in place of the cauliflower, 1 leek and 1 carrot.

Topping
150 g/5 oz wholemeal flour
100 g/3 oz oatbran
1 egg, beaten
50 g/2 oz low-fat cheese, grated
½ tsp baking powder
25 g/1 oz butter

salt and pepper
2 tbsp natural yoghurt

Preheat oven to 180°C/350°F/gas mark 4.

1 Cook carrots and cauliflower in boiling water for 5 minutes. Drain and place in a dish with the sweetcorn.
2 Gently fry the leeks in butter, stirring continually.
3 Melt the butter and stir in the cornflour to make a roux. Remove from the heat, slowly blend in the stock and add the seasoning.
4 Boil, then simmer for 3 minutes. Add the chopped parsley. Place all the vegetables in a casserole dish and pour the sauce over the top. Bake in the oven for 20 minutes.
5 For the scones, rub the butter into the sieved flour, add the bran, cheese and baking powder, saving a little cheese.
6 Add the beaten egg and the yoghurt to form a dough.
7 Roll out and cut into small scones,
8 Arrange over the vegetables and sprinkle on the rest of the cheese. Bake for 15 minutes at 200°C/400°F/gas mark 6 until golden.
If using meat, at stage 2 gently stir fry the meat with the leeks for 5 minutes. Continue as given.

Serve with potatoes mashed together with turnips, approx.⅔ potatoes, ⅓ turnips.

DAY 26

Peppered Fish with Coriander and Lime

Serves 4

2 large white fish fillets (e.g. plaice, lemon sole, Dover sole or halibut)
1 tsp mixed peppercorns, crushed
1 tbsp plain flour
salt and pepper
1 dstsp olive oil
1 clove garlic
2 tsp coarse grain mustard
rind and juice of 2 limes
1 tbsp freshly chopped coriander leaves

1 Mix together the crushed peppercorns, the salt and pepper, and the flour. Skin the fish and press them into the mixture to cover both sides.
2 Crush the garlic and add the mustard, lime juice and rind.
3 Gently heat the olive oil and a dessertspoon of water in a pan and fry the fish for 6–8 minutes, turning once.
4 Add the garlic and lime mixture, using a brush to paste it over the fish and coriander. Cook gently for a further 2–3 minutes.

Serve with new potatoes and a green salad.

DAY 27

Chicken or Vegetable Jalfrezi

Serves 4

400 g/14 oz root vegetables, e.g. carrots, parsnips, swede
25 g/1 oz mangetout, green beans or whole baby sweetcorn
1 dstsp olive oil and the same of water
1 tsp cumin seeds, crushed
1 piece fresh root ginger (approx. 2½ cm/1 inch), grated
1–2 cloves garlic
1 tsp turmeric
2 tsp garam masala
2 dstsps curry paste
2 fresh green chillis, finely chopped
1 red pepper, chopped
12 small or cherry tomatoes, cut in half
28 ml/1 fl. oz coconut milk
1 tbsp chopped coriander
2 bananas, chopped
Meat Option: Replace 200 g/7 oz of the root vegetables with 2 chicken fillets, chopped.

1. Peel and chop the vegetables, and place in boiling water. Boil for 5–6 minutes and drain, saving the water for stock.
2. Gently heat the oil and water in a large pan. Cook the cumin seeds, together with the garlic,

for 1 minute. Add the ginger and cook gently for another minute.

3 Mix the turmeric with the curry paste and a splash of water, and stir in to the mixture.
4 Add the part-cooked vegetables and cook over a gentle heat for 12–15 minutes. Add a little of the stock if necessary.
5 Add the chillis, pepper and tomatoes and continue to cook gently for about 8 minutes. Gradually pour in the coconut milk.
6 Add the mangetout or sweetcorn and chopped bananas.
7 Add the garam masala and coriander and continue to stir for about 5 minutes.
If you are using chicken, add after stage 3 and continue as given.

Serve with rice and low-fat yoghurt with chopped cucumber.

DAY 28

Chick Pea or Chick Pea and Chicken Casserole

Serves 4

1 large onion, chopped
2 cloves garlic, chopped
1 large tin chopped tomatoes
1 425 g/15 oz tin chick peas, drained and rinsed
400 g/14 oz fresh vegetables of your choice, e.g. carrots, courgettes, broccoli, swede, etc.
600 ml/1 pint vegetable stock

2 tbsp fresh parsley
1 tsp thyme and 1 tsp rosemary
1 dstsp tomato purée
salt and pepper
1 dstsp olive oil and the same of water
Meat Option: Replace 150 g/5 oz of the vegetables with 2 chicken fillets, diced.

Preheat oven to 190°C/375°F/gas mark 5.

1 Gently heat the oil and water and fry the onion and garlic for 2 minutes.
2 Add the tomatoes and the vegetables, and stir fry for about 3–4 minutes, then add the tomato purée and mix in well.
3 Add half the stock and boil gently for 1 minute. Add chick peas, herbs and seasoning.
4 Transfer to an ovenproof dish and place in the oven for 20–5 minutes. If preferred, cover and simmer on the hob for 20 minutes.
If you are using meat, add the chicken after stage 1 and continue as given.

Serve with rice or a large jacket potato and grilled tomatoes and mushrooms.

THE END!

Actually it is really the beginning, the beginning of your new lifestyle diet that will help you to tone up, lose weight and change shape. By now, if you have followed the spring clean and the 28-day diet, you will have already seen a difference.

I have given you all the information you need to succeed with your programme and reach your goals. Now it's up to you! You can choose how 'strict' you want to be, but choose a level that you can maintain. Remember, this is all about making long-term changes – for good.

I know that you can achieve a steady and long-lasting rate of weight loss by following this programme. I know that you will become healthier and have more energy – and probably save on your shopping bills too!

I hope you have enjoyed the book, and have found the information helpful and motivating. There is quite a lot to take in, but you should dip into it from time to time, to remind yourself of certain aspects or to help with motivation. I have enjoyed writing it, as I know it can help you to achieve your goals. I wish you success. Good luck!

Index